BACTERIOLOGY RESEARCH DEVELOPMENTS

METHICILLIN-RESISTANT *STAPHYLOCOCCUS AUREUS* (MRSA)

SIGNS, SYMPTOMS AND TREATMENT

BACTERIOLOGY RESEARCH DEVELOPMENTS

Additional books and e-books in this series can be found on Nova's website under the Series tab.

BACTERIOLOGY RESEARCH DEVELOPMENTS

METHICILLIN-RESISTANT *STAPHYLOCOCCUS AUREUS* (MRSA)

SIGNS, SYMPTOMS AND TREATMENT

ERICK PEREIRA ALVES
EDITOR

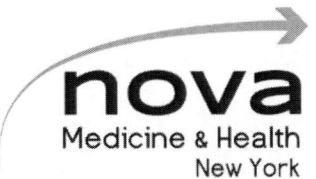

Copyright © 2020 by Nova Science Publishers, Inc.

All rights reserved. No part of this book may be reproduced, stored in a retrieval system or transmitted in any form or by any means: electronic, electrostatic, magnetic, tape, mechanical photocopying, recording or otherwise without the written permission of the Publisher.

We have partnered with Copyright Clearance Center to make it easy for you to obtain permissions to reuse content from this publication. Simply navigate to this publication's page on Nova's website and locate the "Get Permission" button below the title description. This button is linked directly to the title's permission page on copyright.com. Alternatively, you can visit copyright.com and search by title, ISBN, or ISSN.

For further questions about using the service on copyright.com, please contact:
Copyright Clearance Center
Phone: +1-(978) 750-8400   Fax: +1-(978) 750-4470   E-mail: info@copyright.com

NOTICE TO THE READER

The Publisher has taken reasonable care in the preparation of this book, but makes no expressed or implied warranty of any kind and assumes no responsibility for any errors or omissions. No liability is assumed for incidental or consequential damages in connection with or arising out of information contained in this book. The Publisher shall not be liable for any special, consequential, or exemplary damages resulting, in whole or in part, from the readers' use of, or reliance upon, this material. Any parts of this book based on government reports are so indicated and copyright is claimed for those parts to the extent applicable to compilations of such works.

Independent verification should be sought for any data, advice or recommendations contained in this book. In addition, no responsibility is assumed by the Publisher for any injury and/or damage to persons or property arising from any methods, products, instructions, ideas or otherwise contained in this publication.

This publication is designed to provide accurate and authoritative information with regard to the subject matter covered herein. It is sold with the clear understanding that the Publisher is not engaged in rendering legal or any other professional services. If legal or any other expert assistance is required, the services of a competent person should be sought. FROM A DECLARATION OF PARTICIPANTS JOINTLY ADOPTED BY A COMMITTEE OF THE AMERICAN BAR ASSOCIATION AND A COMMITTEE OF PUBLISHERS.

Additional color graphics may be available in the e-book version of this book.

Library of Congress Cataloging-in-Publication Data

Names: Alves, Erick Pereira, editor. Title: Methicillin-resistant *Staphylococcus aureus* (MRSA) : signs, symptoms and treatment / Erick Pereira Alves, editor. Description: New York : Nova Science Publishers, [2020] | Series: Bacteriology research developments | Includes bibliographical references and index. | Summary: "This compilation provides a compact overview of the feasibility and clinical impact of novel therapies for methicillin-resistant *Staphylococcus aureus* (MRSA), with a focus on monoclonal antibodies, vaccines, bacteriophages, liposomes and nanotechnology, photodynamic therapy, homeopathy and botanical medicine. The authors also explore new therapeutic approaches that demonstrate efficacy in scientific research and generate interest in the medical area. Treating nosocomial MRSA infections is challenging due to inadequacies in current therapeutic options and underlying comorbidities in the patients. As such, an overview of the signs, symptoms and treatment options for clinically significant MRSA infections is presented. In closing, the authors examine the occurrence of MRSA in healthcare settings, as well as community-based infections"-- Provided by publisher.
Identifiers: LCCN 2020028352 (print) | LCCN 2020028353 (ebook) | ISBN 9781536181890 (paperback) | ISBN 9781536182699 (adobe pdf)
Subjects: LCSH: *Staphylococcus aureus* infections--Diagnosis. | *Staphylococcus aureus* infections--Treatment. | Methicillin resistance.
Classification: LCC RC116.S8 M49 2020 (print) | LCC RC116.S8 (ebook) | DDC 616.9/297--dc23
LC record available at https://lccn.loc.gov/2020028352
LC ebook record available at https://lccn.loc.gov/2020028353

Published by Nova Science Publishers, Inc. † New York

CONTENTS

Preface		vii
Chapter 1	New Complementary and Alternative Therapies to Control Methicillin-Resistant *Staphylococcus aureus* (MRSA) Infection *Susana Nogueira Diniz, Tânia Aguiar Passeti, Audrey de Souza Marquez, Everton Tadeu Prado, Claudia Forlin da Silva, Danielli dos Santos Baeta and Katia Sivieri*	1
Chapter 2	Methicillin-Resistant *Staphylococcus aureus*: Old and New Therapeutic Approaches *Sandrelli Meridiana de Fátima Ramos dos Santos Medeiros, Iago Dillion Lima Cavalcanti, Ketly Rodrigues Barbosa dos Anjos, Mariane Cajubá de Britto Lira Nogueira and Isabella Macário Ferro Cavalcanti*	79
Chapter 3	MRSA Infections and Treatment: Scope for Options *Hariharan Periasamy and Gnanamani Arumugam*	121

Chapter 4	An Overview on Pathogenesis and Treatment of Methicillin-Resistant *Staphylococcus aureus* (MRSA) *Ritika Chauhan and Jayanthi Abraham*	**155**
Index		**185**

PREFACE

This compilation provides a compact overview of the feasibility and clinical impact of novel therapies for methicillin-resistant *Staphylococcus aureus* (MRSA), with a focus on monoclonal antibodies, vaccines, bacteriophages, liposomes and nanotechnology, photodynamic therapy, homeopathy and botanical medicine.

The authors also explore new therapeutic approaches that demonstrate efficacy in scientific research and generate interest in the medical area.

Treating nosocomial MRSA infections is challenging due to inadequacies in current therapeutic options and underlying comorbidities in the patients. As such, an overview of the signs, symptoms and treatment options for clinically significant MRSA infections is presented.

In closing, the authors examine the occurrence of MRSA in healthcare settings, as well as community-based infections.

Chapter 1 - Methicillin-Resistant *Staphylococcus aureus* (MRSA) became a major public health concern worldwide. The increase in the prevalence of antibiotic resistant pathogens, the limited efficacy and the adverse events associated with antibiotics have urged the development of complementary and alternative methods to treat *Staphylococcus aureus* (*S. aureus*) infections. This chapter provides a compact overview of the feasibility and clinical impact of novel therapies, with a focus on monoclonal antibodies (mAbs), vaccines, bacteriophages, liposomes and nanotechnology, photodynamic therapy (PDT), homeopathy and botanical medicine. Clinical trials with mAbs carried out in subjects with staphylococcal infections demonstrated that the majority failed to prove the efficacy and only a few remain in clinical development. Vaccines targeting *S. aureus* have recently been tested in clinical trials and although the results seem promising, there is currently no vaccine which has proven to be clinically effective. Several case studies have demonstrated the use of bacteriophages to treat infections caused by *S. aureus*. Although this kind of treatment demonstrated to be safe and effective, trials involving a larger population are necessary prior to confidently implement bacteriophages into clinical use. The potential use of liposomal compounds for the treatment of staphylococcal infections and to encapsulate antimicrobial agents as delivery methods, has recently emerged. Results showed that the application of liposomes improves the stability of antimicrobial agents and extends the length of activity, being a promising formulation for bacteria targeted delivery and immune system defense. Antibacterial PDT is a new non-antibiotic treatment strategy for a variety of drug-resistant bacteria including MRSA. Findings on recent studies suggest that PDT can effectively inhibit MRSA by damaging cell membrane, cytoplasm, proteins and nucleic acid. The study of plant extracts with antimicrobial activity allows the identification of active molecules and their mechanism of action, which increases the likelihood of new antimicrobial drugs development or their use in association with known antibiotics to enhance antimicrobial activity. Finally, homeopathic treatment may improve the clinical condition of patients, reduce the need for conventional antimicrobial agents and decrease the relapse rate of infection. Promising results have been obtained with the use of Belladona and MRSA isotherapic to inhibit MRSA growth *in vitro*, suggesting that this phenomenon was not due to bacterial cell death, but rather to a marked decrease in its growth rate, which probably make the bacteria more sensitive to oxacillin. As discussed in this chapter, there are several promising new complementary and alternative therapeutics towards MRSA that may be successfully used in combination with the available conventional antibimicrobial treatments.

Chapter 2 - *Staphylococcus aureus* is a microorganism that presents several virulence factors besides the ability to acquire resistance to a large number of antibiotics. The clinical and indiscriminate use of methicillin allowed the appearance of methicillin-resistant *S. aureus* (MRSA), considered one of the leading causes of nosocomy infections, with high mortality rates worldwide. The pattern of antimicrobial susceptibility and the prevalence of this pathogen varies widely between countries and regions. Infections caused by this microorganism result in a hospital stay increase and high costs associated with medical care. Also, infections caused by MRSA that were previously associated only with hospital environments can already be found in the community infecting people without predisposing risk factors. Therefore, MRSA is not only seen as a nosocomial pathogen. Besides, the prevalence and epidemiology of MRSA are continually changing, with new MRSA strains appearing in different geographic regions. Regarding the therapy, vancomycin has been historically the standard drug for treatment, and sometimes the last resort for the treatment of severe MRSA infections, providing empirical coverage and definitive treatment. However, its indiscriminate use led to the development of vancomycin-resistant *S. aureus* (VRSA). In this sense, this book chapter seeks to describe the main available therapeutic possibilities for the treatment of MRSA/VRSA infections and the new therapeutic approaches that demonstrate efficacy in scientific research and arouse interest in the medical area.

Chapter 3 - Methicillin-resistant *Staphylococcus aureus* (MRSA) are those *S. aureus* isolates carrying a resistance gene *mecA* in their chromosome. Compared to methicillin-susceptible *S. aureus* isolates, MRSA are dreaded as they are resistant to multiple class of antibiotics and only a limited treatment options exist. The MRSA clones cause diverse range of infections both in community and hospitals. These infections include self-resolving skin infections such as impetigo and life-threatening infections such as bacteremia and pneumonia. The ability of MRSA to establish recalcitrant infections is attributed to expression of battery of virulence factors. Management of community MRSA infections is challenging owing to limited MRSA-active oral antibiotic options. Treating nosocomial MRSA infections is much more challenging due to inadequacies in current therapeutic options and underlying comorbidities in the patients. In this chapter, an overview of signs, symptoms and treatment options for clinically important MRSA infections is presented.

Chapter 4 - *Staphylococcus* is a natural inhabitant of the skin and nasal cavities of almost 30 percent of the healthy population. The *Staphylococcus* strains which have developed resistance towards penicillin-related drugs such as amoxicillin and methicillin are known as methicillin-resistant *Staphylococcus aureus* (MRSA). The emergence and various outbreaks of MRSA over the decades have made it difficult to combat antibiotic resistance with the current class of antibiotics. The major causes for prevalence of MRSA are the increasing hospital-associated bacterial infections (HA-MRSA), health care associated MRSA-patients with ongoing dialysis or chemotherapy and also community associated MRSA-transfer from human to human transmission. The present book chapter emphasizes the occurrence of MRSA in health care settings as well as community-based infections, the symptoms and diagnosis associated with MRSA infections, treatment and various mechanisms to combat methicillin resistant *Staphylococcus aureus*.

In: Methicillin-Resistant Staphylococcus ...   ISBN: 978-1-53618-189-0
Editor: Erick Pereira Alves   © 2020 Nova Science Publishers, Inc.

Chapter 1

NEW COMPLEMENTARY AND ALTERNATIVE THERAPIES TO CONTROL METHICILLIN-RESISTANT *STAPHYLOCOCCUS AUREUS* (MRSA) INFECTION

Susana Nogueira Diniz[1,*], *PhD,*
Tânia Aguiar Passeti[1], *PhD,*
Audrey de Souza Marquez[2], *PhD,*
Everton Tadeu Prado[1], *Claudia Forlin da Silva*[1],
Danielli dos Santos Baeta[3] *and Katia Sivieri*[4], *PhD*

[1]Department of Pharmacy and Biotechonology and Health Innovation, Anhanguera University of São Paulo, São Paulo, SP, Brazil
[2]Center of Research in Health Sciences, Unopar University, Londrina, PR, Brazil and Professional Master's Program in Pharmacy, Anhanguera University of São Paulo, São Paulo, SP, Brazil
[3]School of Pharmaceutical Sciences, São Paulo State University, Araraquara, SP, Brazil

---

* Corresponding Author's E-mail: dinizsusana@gmail.com.

[4]Department of Biotechonology and Health Innovation, Anhanguera University of São Paulo, São Paulo, SP, Brazil and School of Pharmaceutical Sciences, São Paulo State University, Araraquara, SP, Brazil

ABSTRACT

Methicillin-Resistant *Staphylococcus aureus* (MRSA) became a major public health concern worldwide. The increase in the prevalence of antibiotic resistant pathogens, the limited efficacy and the adverse events associated with antibiotics have urged the development of complementary and alternative methods to treat *Staphylococcus aureus* (*S. aureus*) infections. This chapter provides a compact overview of the feasibility and clinical impact of novel therapies, with a focus on monoclonal antibodies (mAbs), vaccines, bacteriophages, liposomes and nanotechnology, photodynamic therapy (PDT), homeopathy and botanical medicine. Clinical trials with mAbs carried out in subjects with staphylococcal infections demonstrated that the majority failed to prove the efficacy and only a few remain in clinical development. Vaccines targeting *S. aureus* have recently been tested in clinical trials and although the results seem promising, there is currently no vaccine which has proven to be clinically effective. Several case studies have demonstrated the use of bacteriophages to treat infections caused by *S. aureus*. Although this kind of treatment demonstrated to be safe and effective, trials involving a larger population are necessary prior to confidently implement bacteriophages into clinical use. The potential use of liposomal compounds for the treatment of staphylococcal infections and to encapsulate antimicrobial agents as delivery methods, has recently emerged. Results showed that the application of liposomes improves the stability of antimicrobial agents and extends the length of activity, being a promising formulation for bacteria targeted delivery and immune system defense. Antibacterial PDT is a new non-antibiotic treatment strategy for a variety of drug-resistant bacteria including MRSA. Findings on recent studies suggest that PDT can effectively inhibit MRSA by damaging cell membrane, cytoplasm, proteins and nucleic acid. The study of plant extracts with antimicrobial activity allows the identification of active molecules and their mechanism of action, which increases the likelihood of new antimicrobial drugs development or their use in association with known antibiotics to enhance antimicrobial activity. Finally, homeopathic treatment may improve the clinical condition of patients, reduce the need for conventional antimicrobial agents and decrease the relapse rate of infection. Promising results have been obtained with the use of Belladona and MRSA isotherapic to inhibit MRSA growth *in vitro*, suggesting that this phenomenon was not due to bacterial cell death, but rather to a marked decrease in its growth rate, which probably make the bacteria more sensitive to oxacillin. As discussed in this chapter, there are several promising new complementary and alternative therapeutics towards MRSA that may be successfully used in combination with the available conventional antibimicrobial treatments.

Keywords: methicillin-resistant *Staphylococcus aureus* (MRSA), complementary and alternative therapies, monoclonal antibodies (mAbs), vaccines, bacteriophages, liposomes, nanotechnology, Photodynamic therapy (PDT), homeopathy, botanical medicine

INTRODUCTION

Complementary and Alternative Medicine (CAM) is the term used to define a variety of health practices that do not integrate the conventional medicine therapies and follow a more holistic frame of health system focused on individual aspects, on the integrality of being and on the prevention of diseases [1, 2].

In recent decades, studies involving CAM have increased greatly. An online database search with the keyword "Complementary and Alternative Medicine" revealed more than 20,000 articles on the subject. Frass et al. 2012 reports that CAM use has increased in several countries between 1990 and 2006, as well as a significant boost in the number of studies that address the subject since 2000 [3]. The use of CAM can be performed in several pathologies, including bacterial infections [4]. Several factors are associated with the use of these therapies in association or not with conventional medicine, such as overall well-being, limitations of allopathic medicine and low cost. Its use among healthy people has also become frequent and applied as prophylactic treatment in various conditions such as rheumatic diseases, acquired immunodeficiency syndrome (AIDS), in pediatrics and even as an adjuvant therapy for the treatment of pain in cancer patients. These applications are mainly due to the noninvasive and non-toxic procedures that consists the CAM therapies [2, 5, 6].

Infectious diseases, especially those caused by bacteria resistant to multiple drugs (MDR), are considered one of the main public health problems worldwide [7]. The emergence of penicillin and the use of antibiotics surely had a positive impact in modern medicine and is considered one of the fundamental reasons for the increase of life expectancy in approximately 30 years after 1940 [7, 8]. However, the massive and indiscriminate use of antibiotics, both in human and animal treatment, led to the serious challenge of current bacterial resistance [9]. According to the World Health Organization (2019) [10], 700,000 people die each year as a result of bacterial resistance and it is estimated that this number will reach 10 million deaths per year by 2050, overlapping the estimated mortality from cancer (8.2 million per year). Infections caused by multidrug-resistant microorganisms increase mortality rates, length of hospital stay, and risk for admission to intensive care. This scenario becomes even worse since a new class of antimicrobials has not been developed in the last 25 years, limiting the treatment options for this type of infection [11]. In 2014, the World Health Organization (WHO) published a Global Report on Antimicrobial Resistance in which is revealed that people with MRSA is 64% more likely to die than those with the non-resistant form of the bacteria [8]. Subsequently, WHO launched a Global Action Plan on Antimicrobial Resistance in which the prevalence, emergence and follow-up of critical multi or pan drug-resistant bacteria is monitored in several countries, including MRSA, through the Global Antimicrobial Resistance Surveillance System (GLASS) [12].

Methicillin-resistant *Staphylococcus aureus* (MRSA) is a Gram-positive bacterium that can cause infections in different organs or body systems and is described as one of the main pathogens causing hospital infections and bacteremia [8]. The first record reporting *S. aureus* resistance to methicillin dates from 1960s, in England [13, 14]. Since then, innumerous outbreaks in hospital, nursing homes and community environments have occurred culminating in its classification as one of the leading causes of healthcare-associated infections, responsible for more than eleven thousand deaths per year only in the United States [15, 16]. After its establishment in the community environment, the effective treatment became increasingly difficult due to the enhancement of drug-resistance to frequently used antimicrobials [8, 17]. Because of the increased resistance to known antibiotics, the limitations of allopathic therapeutic options and efficacy, and the adverse events associated with conventional medicine, the complementary and alternative methods become a good option of treatment and play an important role in controlling and fighting of these infections.

For a better understanding of the therapies in the treatment of MRSA infections, it is important to recognize the main virulence factors of the bacterium, which are involved in almost all processes from colonization to host dissemination. They promote adherence to the components of the host's extracellular matrix, damaging its cells and influencing the interaction with the immune system. This interaction defines the possible outcomes of the infection. The bacterium produces an extensive variety of virulence factors with the main objective of evading the host immune responses, which causes cell lysis, tissue invasion and destruction, inhibition of complement activation and the inhibition of phagocytes by the prevention of neutrophils function and recruitment. Those virulence factors can be grouped in types, such as MAMPs (microorganism-associated molecular pattern), adhesins, evasins and toxins. Evasins and toxins represent the majority of *S. aureus* virulence factors. The most prominent ones and their corresponding host ligands were presented in a recent review by Lee et al. 2018 [18]. Figure 1 shows a schematic representation of *S. aureus* most frequent components and virulence factors involved in the development of possible treatments and prevention strategies.

Additionally, the bacteria present virulence systems of defense: the *agr* Operon and the Two-Component System (TCS) [19]. The first consists of a cluster of genes that regulates the decrease or increase in some virulence factors expression, as SEs, hemolysins, capsular polysaccharides (CPs) and proteases, by means of two RNAs (RNA II and RNA III). Although there is evidence of agr operon functions and certain pathogenic outcomes, further studies are necessary to determine clearer connections. The TCS is one of the primary ways the bacteria sense the environment, by a kinase signaling and a response regulator from *agr* system that binds to DNA. This bacteria virulence system promotes the evasion from host innate immune response by reducing reactive oxygen species, the reduction of IL-8 and the increase in leukocidins expression. [19, 20].

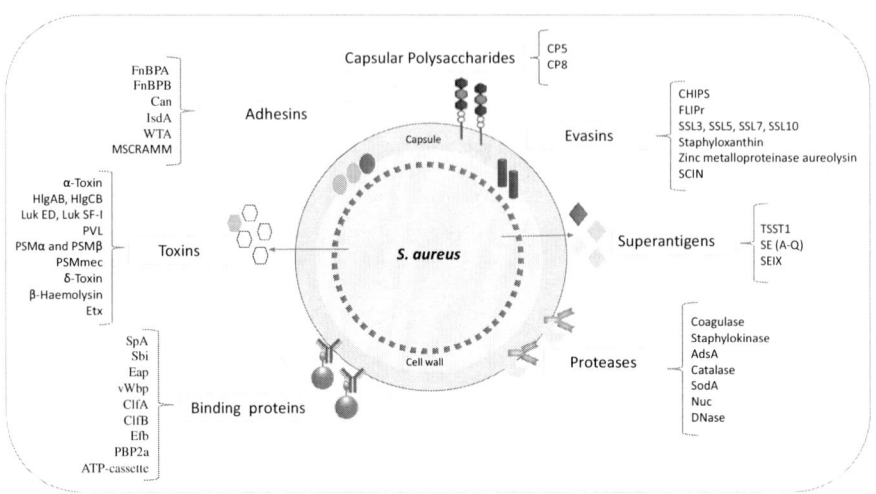

Figure 1. The main virulence factors of *S. aureus* that may function as targets for biological agents. The described factors do not exhaust all those reported in literature. Legend: CP5/CP8 (capsular polysaccharides 5 and 8), CHIPS (chemotaxis inhibitory protein of *S. aureus*), FLIPr (formyl-peptide receptor(FPR)-like 1 inhibitory protein), SSL3/SSL5/SSL7/SSL10 (Staphylococcal superantigen-like proteins), SCIN (Staphylococcal complement inhibitors), TSST1 (Toxic shock syndrome toxin 1), SE (A-Q) (Staphylococcal Enterotoxins types A-Q), SEIX (Staphylococcal enterotoxin-like X), AdsA (Adenosine synthase), SodA (Superoxide dismutase [Mn]), Nuc (Thermonuclease), SpA (Staphylococcus protein A), Sbi (Immunoglobulin-binding protein), Eap (Extracellular adherence protein), vWbp (secreted von-Willebrand factor binding protein), ClfA/ClfB (clumping factor A and B), Efb (fibrinogen-binding protein), HlgAB/HlgCB (Bi-component γ-Haemolysin AB and CB), Luk ED/Luk SF-I (leukocidins ED and SF-I), PVL (Panton–Valentine leukocidin), PSMα/PSMβ (Pore-forming peptide toxins alfa and beta), PSMmec (SCCmec-encoded PSM), Etx (Exfoliative toxins), FnBPA/FnBPB (Fibronectin-binding protein A and B), Can (collagen adhesin), IsdA (iron-regulated surface determinant protein A), WTA (Wall teichoic acid).

Amongst the available options of complementary and alternative treatments to the use of antibiotics, it can be mentioned the use of monoclonal antibodies, active vaccines and bacteriophages, liposomes and nanotechnology, photodynamic therapies, homeopathy and botanical medicine. CAM treatments can be applied when antibiotic therapy is not indicated, helping to reduce the excessive use of antibiotics. MacKay et al.

2003 already suggested the prescription of CAM for pediatric patients, with the main purpose of reducing the use of antibiotics and changing the paradigm with emphasis on patient education, disease prevention and the immune system stimulation, in more accurate diagnosis and the use of simple therapies [4, 19].

In this context, the discovery of monoclonal antibodies (MAbs) and vaccines introduced new approaches for the treatment of various pathologies, including bacterial infections. Studies in mice have shown that a MAb against multi-modular class B penicillin-binding protein (PBP2a) provides protection against MRSA infections, as well as the combination of MAb with vancomycin, which produced greater protection, and the use of staphylococcal antigens as active vaccines that can be effective in the protection of potential *S. aureus* infection [21, 22, 23, 24, 25].

Moreover, bacteriophage therapy is a promising treatment against bacterial infections. Studies show that commercial bacteriophages can attack only pathogenic bacteria without affecting the protective gut microbiota [26, 27]. As an alternative therapy one can also find the combination of antimicrobials with liposomes, which greatly favors the drug antimicrobial activity against the pathogen and attenuates the virulence of the bacterium [28, 29, 30].

Photodynamic therapy (PDT) has also been studied as a promising treatment. When combined with a LED lightv or laser, the dye as photosensitizer contributes to the healing process and tissue repair, along with the bacteriostatic and/or bactericidal activity [31, 32]. A study by Huang et al., 2019, showed that the use of PDT associated with 5-aminolevulinic acid may result in bactericidal effect [33].

The homeopathy, developed by Hahnemann in the 18th century, has as its principle the recovery of individual health using medications prepared in infinitesimal and dynamic dilutions of the active ingredient or therapeutic substance [34]. It presents a fundamental scientific characteristic due to its tradition of evidencing empirical studies with a vast literature of cases and practice reports [35, 36]. Passeti et al. 2016 reported the inhibition of MRSA growth in in vitro tests with Belladona and isotherapic homeopathy medicines, that also enhanced the strain susceptibility to antimicrobial action [37].

Therefore, the research and development of CAM therapies offer the clinician additional options to treat MRSA infections and can be combined with current conventional treatments to provide greater protection to human health. In this chapter some of these therapies will be addressed, as well as future perspectives for the treatment and prevention of MRSA infections.

MONOCLONAL ANTIBODIES

Antibodies are serum immunoglobulins (Igs) that have specific binding affinity to antigens. Monoclonal antibodies (MAbs) are those produced by a single clone of B cells [38]. Köhler and Milstein 1975 discovered that B cells can be immortalized by its fusion with myeloma cells, resulting in hybridoma cells that are able to produce virtually unlimited quantities of monoclonal antibodies [39]. The process of MAb development includes the following successive working phases: the generation of antigen-specific B cells (step 1), the fusion of these cells with myeloma cells (step 2), the cloning and selection of the specific hybridoma clone by "limiting dilution" (step 3) and the up-scaling of MAb production (step 4) (Figure 2) [40]. Since the Nobel price-winning work of these researchers (1984), MAbs have become essential tools in basic research as well as in diagnostic testing and medical treatments, including infectious diseases. Usually, therapeutic MAbs are developed and directed against non-human targets, virulent factors or toxins, in order to neutralize microorganism virulence activity, rendering it as nonpathogenic, while blocking the bacterium's mechanisms for escaping immune response [41]. MAbs are fast acting drugs and have shown to be effective, but the biggest challenge of this therapy is to find pathogens molecular determinants that are accessible on the cell surface and to modulate elements of the host immune system.

Staphylococcus aureus (S. aureus) possesses an elaborate resource of virulence factors that serve as targets for the development of anti-staphylococcal MAbs (Figure 1). Considering the complexity of its virulence system, it is highly recommended that MAbs for the treatment of *S. aureus* should be: multi-valent agents and designed to target the bacterium's elaborate extracellular and intracellular antigens, able to neutralize virulence factors, and able to target elements of the host immune system, in an effort to boost or restore host immunity, enhance phagocytosis and complement activation, as well as induce immunoglobulin isotype-dependent actions [42, 43, 25, 44].

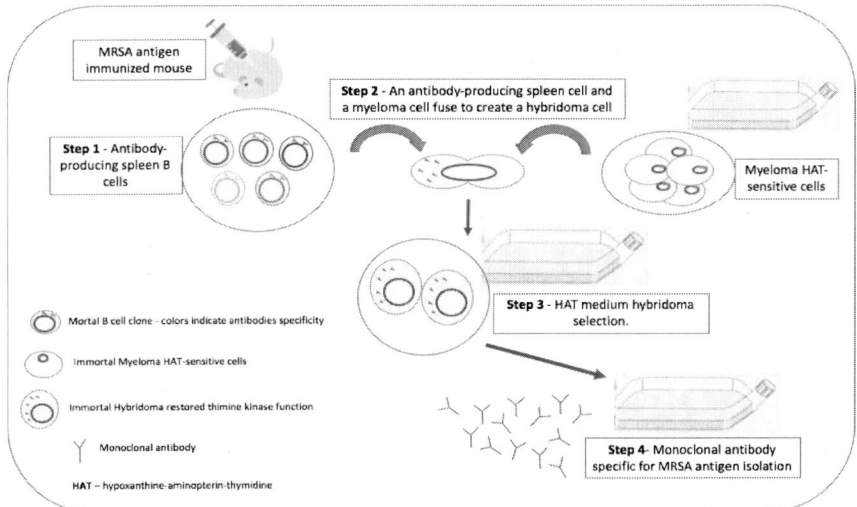

Figure 2. The production of Monoclonal antibodies. Step1 - Generation of antigen-specific B cells by injection of MRSA antigen in mice and isolation of spleen cells, including those that produce antibodies. Different antibody colors indicate antibodies specific for different molecules (antigens) produced by different cells. Step 2 - The fusion of antibody-producing spleen of limited lifespan with myeloma cells, an immortal antibody-secreting immune cell of unknown specificity, generating hybrid cells called hybridomas. Step 3 - Cloning and Selection of specific hybridomas. HAT selection depicted by a myeloma thymidine kinase mutant fused with a mortal splenic B-cell. Unlike unfused cells, the hybridoma cells could grow on the selective medium and form colonies of identical cells. Step 4 - Up-scaling of MAbs production. Hybridomas that secreted antibodies specific for MRSA were identified by their ability to bind or destroy that bacteria.

In addition, the use of monoclonal antibodies together with antibiotic has been proposed as a promising strategy for the restraint of MDR bacteria, as MAbs treatment should potentiate antibiotic effectiveness. The inclusion of MAb therapies in this chapter has the purpose of offering hope in the prevention and/or treatment of severe and invasive disease, for which antibiotic therapy is too often insufficient, such as in MRSA infections. Efforts to treat infections with MAbs targeting *S. aureus* extracellular and intracellular components or elements from host immunity have been evaluated in preclinical and clinical trials. In general, MAbs have shown to be effective to treat *S. aureus* infection in immunocompromised mice [45], have an excellent safety record [46, 47] and, like other alternative therapies, can complement antibiotic therapy, showing the effectiveness of the association of MAbs with antimicrobial agents [46, 48, 49, 50]. Although these trials have made progress in proving the clinical safety of mAbs, and concluded that the antibodies tested could ultimately treat or protect patients infected or at risk of infection by this MDR bacterium, the efficacy of these drugs in reducing pathogenesis is yet to be proven. The main studies are subsequent described.

Recent preclinical studies developed three human monoclonal antibodies against all F-components of hemolysin HlgAB/CD, leukocidins LukSF, and LukED. These antibodies were found to be capable of blocking leukocidin-mediated rabbit red blood cell lysis *in vitro* and significantly reduced disease progression and mortality after murine peritonitis by *S. aureus* infection, *in vivo* [43]. A recent study evaluated MAbs against the PBP2a, a multi-modular class B penicillin-binding protein (PBP), located external to the membrane of all MRSA strains. The authors demonstrated that MAb confers MRSA protection in a murine model both as prophylactic, by reducing bacterial load, and therapeutic treatment, by increasing survival rate in treated mice. The results suggest that MAbs directed against PBP2a are a promising approach for treating infections caused by MRSA strains [25]. Another study showed the isolation of human monoclonal antibody anti-exotoxin staphylococcal enterotoxin B (SEB), designated as M0313, that was efficient to inhibit SEB-induced proliferation of mouse splenic lymphocyte and human peripheral blood mononuclear cells, and to inhibit cytokine release in cell culture. M0313 also neutralized SEB toxicity in BALB/c female mice and promoted the survival of mice infected with SEB-expressing bacteria [44].

Tefibazumab is a humanized monoclonal antibody to *S. aureus* adhesins MSCRAMM (acronym for "microbial surface components recognizing adhesive matrix molecules"). Clinical trials demonstrated that Veronate™, a biologic agent containing MAb tefibazumab that targets *S. aureus* clumping factor A (ClfA,), was evaluated as an adjunctive therapy to antibiotic treatment in *S. aureus* bacteremia patients [51]. This MAb was also shown to protect rabbits from *S. aureus* infection and demonstrated opsonophagocytic activity [52]. Tefibazumab was shown to be tolerated well in a Phase II trial focused on safety and pharmacokinetics [53, 54]. A Phase III, Randomized, Double-blind, Multi-center Clinical Trial Comparing the Safety and Efficacy of Veronate® Versus Placebo for the Prevention of Nosocomial Staphylococcal Sepsis in Premature Infants was developed and showed promising results [55, 56]. However, Tefibazumab producers suspended indefinitely the pending trials due to licensing negotiations.

Aurexis is a humanized monoclonal antibody containing tefibazumab, for the treatment of severe *S. aureus* infections. A Phase IIa dose escalation study to assess safety and pharmacokinetics of Aurexis® in cystic fibrosis subjects chronically colonized with *S. aureus* in their lungs, demonstrated that this biological agent is safe regarding the concentration of Aurexis in blood and sputum [57]. Another trial with this monoclonal antibody was developed with the purpose of assessing the safety and pharmacokinetics of standard antibiotic therapy, plus Aurexis or Placebo, for the treatment of *S. aureus* bacteremia (SAB). The authors did not show any benefit to these patients [58].

Pagibaximab, also named BS4X, a mAb that targets lipoteichoic acid (WTA), a key component of the bacterial Gram-positive cell wall, was shown to enhance opsonophagocytosis of *S. epidermidis*. The clinical trial Phase I of BSYX-A110, a human chimeric anti-Staphylococcal monoclonal antibody, in adults, demonstrated the prevention of *S. epidermidis* infection in low birth weight infants [59, 60]. Phase IIb/III, randomized, double-blind, multicenter, placebo-controlled study evaluate the safety, efficacy and pharmacokinetics (PK) of pagibaximab for the prevention of staphylococcal sepsis in low birth weight infants. The subjects were monitored for adverse events and tolerability to drug infusion. Neonatal sepsis was assessed in the presence of clinical signs and symptoms and one blood culture positive for *S. aureus* or two blood cultures positive for Coagulase-Negative Staphylococci [61, 62]. Despite promising results for the prevention of *S. aureus* sepsis in low birth weight neonates, in Phase II, Pagibaximab ultimately failed in a more comprehensive Phase III sepsis trial [63, 64].

The single-chain mAb fragment, Aurograb, targets *S. aureus* ATP-binding cassette (ABC) transporter. This molecule was selected from an innovative screen that identified immunodominant antigens in the sera of septic patients [48]. The response to Aurograb® (1mg/kg i.v. b.d.) plus vancomycin is greater than the overall response to placebo plus vancomycin, in patients with severe, deep-seated staphylococcal infections. While Aurograb demonstrated to work synergistically with vancomycin to reduce *S. aureus* burden in the organs of infected mice, the drug was shown to be ineffective in a Phase III trial [48, 65, 49, 50]. For note, no peer-reviewed preclinical data has been made available for Aurograb.

Clinical trials have also been conducted on mAbs targeting toxins which are unique to *S aureus* [45, 46, 47, 41]. In the study of Rouha et al. (2018), ASN100 is used as a combination of two mAbs: ASN1 (targeting alpha-toxin and four of the five hemolysins: HlgAB, HlgCB, LukED, LukSFPV) and ASN2 (targeting LukGH) in a Phase II study. Results demonstrated that syncytial use of both mAbs, *in vitro*, blocked the cytolytic activity of *S. aureus* [41]. However, a Phase II clinical study with ASN100 in mechanically ventilated patients at risk for S aureus pneumonia was recently halted as it was not likely to meet the primary end-point. [66].

Suvratoxumab, another MAb named MEDI4893, is an extended half-life human monoclonal antibody against *Staphylococcus aureus* alpha-toxin was evaluated in clinical trial to analyze safety, tolerability and pharmacokinetics [46, 67, 68].

Another MAb KBSA301, known as AR-301 or Salvecin, is a fully human monoclonal antibody that binds to Staphylococcal alpha-toxin. The objectives of this study are to assess the safety, tolerability, pharmacokinetics, pharmacodynamics and clinical outcome of patients who have severe pneumonia caused by *S. aureus* after a single intravenous administration of KBSA301 in association with antibiotic [47, 68].

A recent trial, randomized, double-blind, placebo-controlled multicenter Phase III study of efficacy and safety of AR-301 as an adjunct therapy to antibiotics in the treatment of ventilator-associated pneumonia (VAP) caused by *S. aureus* is evaluating the cure rate by measuring the need for mechanical ventilation and signs and symptoms of pneumonia [69, 70].

The MAb 514G3 targets the surface antigen Staphylococcal protein A (SpA), which also aids bacterial clearance. Its mechanism of action focuses on inducing opsonophagocytosis and on inhibiting the immune evasion mechanisms of *S aureus*. It was showed that healthy humans have neutralizing anti-SpA antibodies. These antibodies, when isolated and cloned into an IgG3 background, are successfully able to bind to MRSA strains via their Fab regions with high affinity, leaving the Fc exposed for opsonophagocytosis. A recent study demonstrated that 514G3 antibodies can successfully rescue mice from MRSA challenge, and can be used either as a mono therapy, or as a co-therapy along with vancomycin [71]. A Phase I study on 16 patients with *S aureus* bacteremia (12 studies and 4 placebo) demonstrated 514G3 to be safe and well tolerated at all dose levels tested [72]. A randomized controlled trial evaluated the efficacy of 514G3 in reducing complications of *S. aureus* bacteremia. Patients will receive 514G3 plus antibiotics or placebo plus antibiotics in approximately a 3 to 1 ratio [73]. The results were not published until now.

A summary of MAbs biological agents evaluated for clinical efficacy against *S. aureus* are show in Table 1. Interesting points have to be identified in this area of therapy: it is common the use of combined therapy with antibiotic for the treatment of MRSA infections, the number of possible combinations is quite high, a number of *in vitro* studies have been performed in this area and the number of studies that have analyzed this topic in the clinical setting of MRSA infections is very limited. Since the discovery of monoclonal antibodies in 1975, researchers have been developing several strategies of application. However, for the treatment of *S. aureus* infections, clinical trials with MAbs demonstrated that the majority failed to prove efficacy and only a few remain in development.

Table 1. Clinical trials of monoclonal antibodies against *S. aureus*

Agent	Sponsor(s)/Investigator	Target	Primary clinical indication	Status	Identifier
Tefibazumab (Veronate, Aurexis)	Bristol-Myers Squibb/Seth V. Hetherington	Adhesins surface protein, clumping factor A (ClfA)	*S. aureus* Bacteremia, Nosocomial Infections, Sepsis, Staphylococcal Infections, Candidemia	Completed	NCT00113191 [56] NCT00198289 [57] NCT00198302 [58]
Pagibaximab (BS4X-A110)	Biosynexus Incorporated/ Leonard Weisman, MD	Lipoteichoicacid (LTA)	Neonatal, Staphylococcal Sepsis, Staphylococcal Sepsis	Completed	NCT00636285 [60] NCT00646399 [62] NCT00631800 [63] NCT00631878 [64]
Aurograb	NeuTec Pharma/Mark H Wilcox	ATP-binding cassette (ABC) Transporter GrfA	Staphylococcal Infections	Completed	NCT00217841 [65]
ASN100 (Mab ASN1 and ASN2)	Arsanis, Inc.	Alpha toxin and leukocidins: HlgAB, HlgCB, LukED, LukSFPV, LukGH	Pneumonia, Ventilator-associated Pneumonia, Staphylococcal	Terminated	NCT02940626 [66]
Suvratoxumab (MEDI4893)	MedImmune LLC/Howard Schwartz, M.D	Alpha toxin	*S. aureus* pneumonia	Completed	NCT01769417 [67] NCT02296320 [68]
KBSA301 (AR-301 or Salvecin)	Aridis Pharmaceuticals, Inc./Pierre-François M Laterre, MD/Lynne M Deans, MT	Alpha toxin	Lung Infection, Pneumonia, Ventilator-Associated, Infection, Bacterial, *S. aureus*	Recruiting	NCT01589185 [69] NCT03816956 [70]
514G3	XBiotech, Inc./Mark Rupp, M.D	Surface antigen Staphylococcal protein A (SpA).	*S. aureus* Bacteremia	Completed	NCT02357966 [73]

VACCINES

Despite numerous attempts and investigations, currently there is no staphylococcal vaccines approved for clinical use [74, 75, 76]. Some of the possible reasons for these failures could be the selection of inappropriate antigens, *S aureus* high antigenic variability and immune evasion mechanisms [77]. The first studies focused on vaccines that induced the production of high titers of opsonic antibodies to single-components of surface antigens of *S. aureus*, such as capsular polysaccharides (mainly CP5 and CP8), followed by targets as the toxins (α-hemolysin, Enterotoxin B, LuKS-PV), adhesion factors (C1Fa, A1f3) or nutrient-scavenging factors (IsdB, MntC, FhuD2). These attempts were based on successful vaccine strategies for other pathogens like *Streptococcus pneumoniae* and *Hemophylus influenza* [78, 79, 80, 81, 82, 83]. Even though some of these experiments could show efficacy on animal models, they have failed to demonstrate effectiveness in human clinical trials Phase II or III [84, 78, 75]. This could be due to MRSA's ability to suppress the immune system response through its virulence factors, the superantigens (SAgs) and pore-forming toxins (PFTs), and the fact that it can evade the defense cells and antibodies in biofilms, intracellular auxotrophic small-colony variants or inside abscesses in which it multiplies and causes persistent infections [85, 86, 87, 88, 89, 76].

Another concern related to the vaccine failing is the reliability of animal models in preliminary clinical trials phases. *S aureus* tend to show limited virulence activity in some animal experiments, especially in murine models, in which the SAgs and PFTs are not fully expressed [90, 91, 92]. Furthermore, it has been reported harmful results in Phase III clinical trial of *S. aureus* vaccine containing nonadjuvanted iron-regulated-surface-determinant-B (IsdB), as it appeared to be associated with multi-organ system failure in postoperative subjects [93]. Table 2 shows recent and undergoing candidates for *S. aureus* active vaccine.

Table 2. Developing active vaccines to prevent *S. aureus* infections

Candidate Vaccine	Developer	Target Antigen(s)	Assessed Immune Response	Research Phase	Status and Results	Reference
5-combo OMV$_{SmsbBpagP}$	N.A.	HlaH35L, SpAKKAA, FhuD2, Csa1A, and LukE	Humoral and cellular	Preclinical	Showed high protection in three relevant mouse models.	Carmela et al. (2019) [94]
N.A.	N.A.	CP5/CP8 (purified, CRM197 conjugated)	Humoral	Preclinical	Completed (elicited protection in mice against bacteremia, but not lethal sepsis; in the skin infection model only conjugated CP8 protected against dermonecrosis)	Cheng et al. (2017) [95]
N.A	NIAID	AT62 (recombinant from Hla)	Humoral	Preclinical	Stopped (scarce control of murine skin infection)	Adhikari et al. (2016) [96]
N.A	Pasture Institute of Iran and IAUPS (Tehran, Iran)	PBP2a (recombinant)	Humoral	Preclinical	Completed (efficacy, reduced mortaliy against bacteriumMRSA infection)	Haghighat et al. (2017) [22 ou 23]
N.A.	N.A.	D-alanine auxotrophic mutant (live mutant bacterium)	Humoral and cellular	Preclinical	Completed (efficacy, reduction of abscesses formation in mice)	Moscoso et al. (2018) [97]
SpA-DKKAAFnB PA37-507 (SF)	NSFC (Beijing, China)	SpA/FnBPA (bivalent fusion vaccine, recombinant proteins)	Humoral and cellular	Preclinical	Completed (efficacy, reduction of pneumonia and skin abscesses in mice)	Yang et al. (2018) [98]
GSK239210 3A	GSK (Novartis) (Siena, Italy)	CP5/CP8/Hla/ClfA (conjugated CP5/CP8 plus recombinant Hla/ClfA)	N.A.	Phase I	Completed (no further development)	Levy et al. (2015) [99]

Candidate Vaccine	Developer	Target Antigen(s)	Assessed Immune Response	Research Phase	Status and Results	Reference
4C-Staph	Novartis (Sien, Italy)	FhiD2, EsxAB, HLa, Sur-2	Humoral and cellular	Preclinical	Completed (efficacy, reduction of murine lung infections and arthritis)	Torre et al. (2015) Mancini et al. (2016) [100, 101]
NDV3	NovaDigm Therapeutics (Grand Forks, North Dakota, USA)	rAls3p-N (C. albicans surface protein cross reacting with S. aureus; alum adjuvated)	Humoral and cellular	Phase I	Completed (safety and immunogenicity, stopped phase II due to enrolment problem)	Schmidt et al. (2012) [102]
SA75	Vaccine Research International (Moseley, Birmingham, UK)	Whole cell vaccine	Humoral and cellular	Phase I	Completed (safety and tolerability, no further development)	Giersing et al. (2016) [81]
N.A.	Integrated BioTherapeutics	Enterotoxins A and C1, TSST (recombinant)	Humoral	Phase I	Completed (safety, evaluating possible phase II trial)	Roetzer et al. (2016) [103]
STEBvax	Integrated BioTherapeutics and NIAID (Rockville, Maryland, USA)	Enterotoxin B (rSEB) (recombinant, alum adjuvated)	Humoral	Phase I	Completed (safety, demonstrated production of toxin neutralizing antibodies)	Chen et al. (2016) [104]
N.A.	Nabi Biopharmaceuticals (Rockville, Maryland, USA)	rAT(α-toxin)/rLukS-PV (recombinant)	Humoral	Phase I	Completed (safety, robust immune response)	Landrum et al. (2017) [105]
SA4AG (PF-06290510)	Pfizer (Pearl River, New York, USA)	4-component CP5/CP8 glycoconjugates/ClfA/Mnt C vaccine	Humoral and cellular	Clinical Phase I and IIa	Completed (safety, robust immune response, ongoing phase IIb in adults undergoing spinal fusion surgery)	Anderson et al. (2012) Creech et al. (2017) Bergier et al. (2016)

Table 2. (Continued)

Candidate Vaccine	Developer	Target Antigen(s)	Assessed Immune Response	Research Phase	Status and Results	Reference
SA4AG (PF-06290510)	Pfizer (Pearl River, New York, USA)	4-component CP5/CP8 glycoconjugates/ClfA/Mnt C vaccine	Humoral and cellular	Clinical Phase IIb	Discontinued (low statistical probability to meet primary efficacy in adults undergoing spinal fusion surgery)	Frenck et al. (2017) [106, 107, 108, 109] Gurtman et al. (2018) [110]
StaphVAX	Nabi Biopharmaceuthicals (Rockville, Maryland, USA)	2-component CP5/CP8 purified and conjugated capsular polysaccharides	Humoral	Clinical Phase III	Stopped (no differences between vaccine and placebo in end-stage renal patients)	Fattom et al. (2015) [92]
V710	Merck (Kenilworth, New Jersey, USA)	single-component IsdB purified surface protein	Humoral	Clinical Phase III	Stopped (increased mortality rate in vaccinated patients' post-cardiothoracic surgery)	Fowler et al. (2013) McNeely et al. (2014) [80, 93]

Source: Adapted from Redi et al. (2018). Legend: GSK: GlaxoSmithKline; CP: capsular polysaccharide antigens; Hla/AT: α-toxin; Clf: clumping factor; Als3p: agglutinin like sequence 3 protein; TSST: toxic shock syndrome toxin; Mnt: manganese transporter protein; LukS-PV: Panton–Valentine leukocidin component S; Isd: iron surface determinant; CRM: cross-reacting mutant, a nontoxic recombinant mutant of diphtheria toxin; PBP: penicillin binding protein; Sdr: serine-aspartate repeat proteins; Fhu: ferric hydroxamate uptake; Esx: secretion system protein; Csa: conserved staphylococcal antigens; Clf: clumping factor; Sp: staphylococcal protein; FnBP: fibronectin-binding protein; NIAID: National Institute of Allergy and Infectious Diseases, USA; IAUPS: Islamic Azad University, Pharmaceutical Sciences Branch; NSFC: National Natural Science Foundation of China; N.A.: not available.

It is important to highlighted that the diverse range of virulence factors and patterns of expression in different geographical *S. aureus* clones hinder the achievement of a successful universal MRSA vaccine [83, 18].

More recent investigations tend to focus on multivalent vaccines, but a better understanding of human immunity against MRSA, as well as the validation of a potential vaccine in *S aureus* carriers before conducting larger clinical trials, is essential for future vaccine development [76, 77, 111].

Several data sources indicate that the neutralization of *S. aureus* superantigens SAgs and PFTs correlates to better outcomes in invasive MRSA infections, once these virulence factors promote an impairment of host immune response. Consequently, to aim in multivalent anti-toxins Staphylococcal vaccine can be a goal in the attempt of reducing complicated and lethal outcomes in severe infections [76, 112, 113]. Moreover, the stimulation of both humoral and cell-mediated immune responses is essential as antibodies play an important role in the protection from circulating bacteria while Th1 and Th17 responses prevent skin abscesses and promote gastrointestinal clearance [114, 115, 116, 117]. A study based on a new approach using outer membrane vehicles (OMVs) to deliver five *S aureus* antigens demonstrated high protection against the infection in three different mouse models and also suggests that for a better efficiency, when the risk of infection is increased as in hospitalization situations, *S aureus* vaccine should be administered repeatedly [94]. Therefore, a vaccine that shows efficacy for MRSA bacteremia may not protect adequately for skin, soft tissues or bone infections.

In addition, host genetic features can influence the bacteria and the immune system interactions, thus meddling the infection outcome and vaccine efficacy [118, 119]. It has been studied the host genetics features in the susceptibility for severe MRSA infections that could, for example, explain disparities in the prevalence of bacteremia amongst African American individuals [120, 121]. Cyr and colleagues discussed the possible association of HLA Class II region in the susceptibility for *S. aureus* bacteremia [122]. Moreover, it has not been established a protective antibody threshold for effective vaccine response. This increases the costs for proof-of-efficacy trials required for vaccine approval by the Food and Drug Administration (FDA) [123].

Regardless the challenges, a protective vaccine against *S. aureus* is an important strategy to prevent MRSA invasive infections, as bacteremia and pneumonia. Furthermore, approximately one third of the worldwide population are carriers of *S. aureus* and potential candidates for complications, [75], in which an efficient vaccine could prevent severe and fatal infections or reduce MRSA colonization, as well as decrease the use of antibiotics.

To date, there is no vaccine available against MRSA. However, more recent investigations tend to focus on multivalent vaccines, but a better understanding of human immunity against MRSA, as well as the validation of a potential vaccines in *S. aureus* carriers patients, before conducting clinical trials, are key steps for development future of the vaccine.

BACTERIOPHAGES

Probably, MRSA strains are the pathogenic bacteria best known to the general public. In addition to its potential to acquire resistance to antibiotics, *S. aureus* can produce a large number of virulence factors (Figure 3), in addition to exhibiting the ability to form biofilms, as well as to evolve into different clones that can spread and colonize new environments [124]. Then, the emergence of life-threatening MRSA has led to increased interest in the use of bacteriophages as an alternative therapy to antibiotics [125].

Bacteriophages are viruses that infect bacteria in a specific species manner, without any damage to human or animal cells. They have a nucleic acid genome that encodes the functions necessary for their replication, but it needs the host cell for its replication. Viruses can only replicate if the virion, a protein envelope that contains the viral genome and penetrates the host cell [126].

The phages can be member of all body niches, such as skin, oral cavity, lungs, gut, and urinary tract. Most phages present in these viromes are temperate phages that can integrate their DNA into the bacterial genomes or be present as episomes, and as such can alter the phenotype of the host bacteria by lysogenic conversion. Although human blood is considered sterile, metagenomic analysis has shown the presence of a viral community. The human gut microbiome, as shown by metagenomic studies, includes many viral genes (the virome). Approximately 90% of the gut virome consists of phages, estimated at 10^9 viruses per gram of feces [127]. In additional, it has also been shown that bacteriophages are part of the innate immune system in the mammalian gut [128].

Bacteriophages are classified according to the morphological type, host, and the type of nucleic acid. They can be either single or double stranded DNA or single or double stranded RNA. Double-stranded phages can be contractile, non-contractile, tailless and pleomorphic with a lipid envelope. Single-stranded phages can be icosahedral or filamentous. Thirteen families and 46 genera of bacteriophages are already known. Double-stranded and tailed phages belong to the order of Caudovirales, which represent 96% of reported phages. The genome of a phage that has a tail includes the genes that encode DNA packaging and replication, transcription regulation, host lysis, head, tail and fimbria formation. The capsid has the function of protecting genetic information and the tail and fimbriae are involved in the binding of the phage to the host bacteria [129].

Once inside the host cells, a viral genome can orchestrate two distinct events. The first one, the virus can replicate and destroy the host (lytic cycle). In a lytic infection, the virus redirects the host's metabolism to support virus replication. Thus, new virions are released, and the process can be repeated in new host cells. However, some viruses can carry out a lysogenic infection; in this case the viral genome integrates into and replicates with the bacterial chromosome. The viral genetic material, known as prophage, can stay in this state for generations until an environmental signal turns on the machinery leading to its excision from the bacterial genome and kick-starts the lytic cycle [130].

The phage infection pathway involves several steps: phage adsorption on the host cell surface, DNA injection into the host, DNA replication, phage particle assembly, and host lysis (Figure 3). Phage adsorption is mediated by phage receptor-binding proteins (RBPs) and receptors on the bacterial cell surface. This step is critical for determining the success of phage infection, as well as the phage's host range [124]. One of the main advantages of using bacteriophages as antimicrobials is their sheer quantity and diversity. As a matter of fact, even without improvement by genetic engineering, nature represents an almost limitless source of new phage variants. It is well known that phages are the most abundant biological entities on earth (about 10^{31} phages in total) [131].

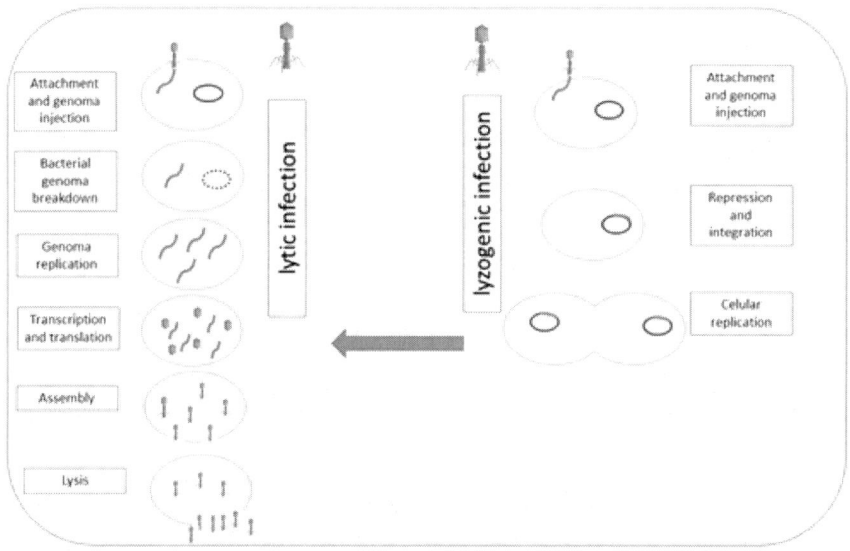

Figure 3. Lytic and lysogenic bacteriophage infection. A bacteriophage infects a bacterial host via genome injection. In the lytic infection the bacterial genome breaks down and the bacteriophage genome replicates, resulting in mature new bacteriophage clones that diffuse through the surrounding environment and they can infect new susceptible bacteria. In lysogenic bacteriophages infection, after injection of the genome, it becomes integrated into a specific section of the bacterial genome and will be replicated every time the bacterial cell duplicates. The bacteriophage genome integrated in the bacterial genome or existing as an extrachromosomal plasmid is called a prophage. Cell divisions produce a population of bacterial cells harboring the bacteriophage genomic material. Environmental factors can induce a lysogenic bacteriophage to enter the lytic cycle. Source: Adapted from Leitner et al. (2019) [129].

Another way for the direct use of phages as antimicrobials is the use of proteins encoded by these agents: endolysins [132]. Lytic phages present a genetic cassette encoding a holin-endolysin system. At the end of the reproductive cycle, once mature viral particles have been assembled, holins are synthesized in critical concentrations and inserted into the cell membrane, creating pores for the translocation of endolysins, previously accumulated in the cytoplasm, to reach the peptidoglycan structure. In additional, endolysins encoded by double-stranded DNA bacteriophages have a molecular weight between 25 and 40 kDa. Most of endolysins are composed of at least two functional domains: one containing the catalytic activity located generally in the N-terminal domain and one responsible for the recognition of a specific substrate associated with the C-terminal domain. In some cases, more than one catalytic domain or more than one recognition domain are present. The recognition domain usually joins to specific molecules in the bacterial cell envelopes such as monosaccharides, coline or teichoic acids. Endolysin activity is usually species specific, although there have been reports of endolysins with a wider substrate range. Besides, the cell wall recognition domain is not always essential for endolysin activity. The endolysin got a wider substrate range, but it conserved certain specificity, since it was not active against all bacteria [133].

The Tables 2 and 3 show the bacteriophages isolated by different sources and its clinical application to control infection by Methicillin-Resistant *Staphylococcus aureus*. In all studies the phages are lytic. The temperate phages are known to actively contribute to the phenomenon of horizontal gene transfer, one of the main mechanisms involved in the spread of antimicrobial resistance and virulence genes [130]. It is important to highlight that are several animal or in vitro studies, but there are few clinical studies. In this context, to get the most out of phage therapy, it will need to have an arsenal of well-chosen effective and safe bacteriophages. The idea of using bacteriophages in clinical therapy is wonderful, but from the initial idea to clinical practice there is a long way. This involves several steps that, if carefully planned, may hinder the successful development and subsequent implementation of this strategy. In additional, before clinical testings, it is particularly important to know if the phage can be propagated in industrial production scale [131].

In conclusion, the phage therapy could help prevent antibiotic resistance, treat resistant infections and reduce antibiotic microbiome injury. Wound infections, especially diabetic foot infections with osteomyelitis, offer an excellent opportunity to demonstrate the potential of phage therapy to heal wounds more quickly and effectively while reducing the harms associated with antibiotics.

Table 3. Bacteriophages targeting Methicillin-Resistant *Staphylococcus aureus* in preclinical studies

Bacteriophages	Type	Source	Therapeutically effective	Reference
AB-SA01	lytic phage	-	Neutropenic and immunocompetent mouse models of acute pneumonia	Lehman et al., 2019 [134]
ϕMR-5 and MR-10 (isolated or in combination)	Lytic phage	Sewage	Decrease of diabetic excision wound infection	Chhibber et al., 2013 [135]
MR-5 and MR-10 (transfersome-entrapped bacteriophage cocktail)	Lytic phage	-	Thigh infections in experimental rats	Chhibber et al., 2017 [136]
ϕSLPW	Lytic phage	Fecal sewage in a pig farm	Decrease of intra-abdominal infection	Wang et al., 2016 [137]
ϕMR-5	Lytic phage	Sewage	Decrease of orthopedic implant infections	Kaur et al., 2016 [138]
SATA-8505 (ATCC PTA-9476)	Lytic phage	-	USA300 infection in human cells *in vitro* and in a mouse model of skin infection	Pincus et al., 2015 [139]
S13'	Lytic phage	Local sewage	Lung-derived septicemia in mouse	Takemura-Uchiyama et al., 2014 [140]
Stau2	Lytic phage	Hospital effluents	Mice infected with *S. aureus* S23 showed that protection by Stau2 from a lethal bacterial infection occurred in a Dose-dependent manner.	Hsieh et al., 2011 [141]
ϕMR11	Lytic phage	-	Control of bacteremia	Matsuzaki et al., 2003 [142]

Table 4. Bacteriophages targeting Methicillin-Resistant *Staphylococcus aureus* in clinical studies

Bacteriophages	Type	Therapeutically effective	Reference
AB-SA01	Lytic phage	Recalcitrant chronic rhinosinusitis	Ooi et al., 2019 [143]
"Phagogram"	Lytic phage	Relapsing prosthetic joint infection	Ferry et al., 2018 [144]
staphylococcal phage Sb-1	Lytic phage	Osteomyelitis in an ulcerated	Fish et al., 2018 [145]
Sb-1	Lytic phage	Diabetic foot ulcer infections	Fish et al., 2016 [146]
SATA-8505 (ATCC PTA-9476)	Lytic phage	Corneal infection	Fadlallah et al., 2015 [147]
polyvalent phage preparation WPP-201	Lytic phage	Venous leg ulcers	Rhoads et al., 2013 [148]
SCCmec type IVc and similar to the OSPC clone	-	Sepsis complicated with severe pneumonia secondary to injury	Gelatti et al., 2009 [149]

LIPOSOME AND NANOTECHNOLOGY

Over the last decade, a significant acceleration in the development of nanotechnology has been observed. The nanomedicine uses nanomaterial platforms for diagnostic and therapeutic procedures enabling the specific drug delivery to target tissues and improving the effectiveness of antimicrobial drugs. In this chapter we will present a brief definition of liposomes and nanotechnology and their benefits as new therapy alternatives for control of MRSA infection.

Liposomes are small vesicles consisting of one or more concentric phospholipid bilayers and spontaneously organize around an aqueous compartment and serve as carriers of biomolecules, drugs, genetic material or diagnostic agents. In aqueous medium the component of the solution used can fill the inside cavity of the liposome, this solution may contain ions or molecules that will organize inside of the liposome [150]. The encapsulation of drugs in liposomes leads to a change in their pharmacokinetic and biodistribution properties, which allow dependence on the physicochemical properties of liposomes, uniformly modifying their original toxicity and therapeutic efficacy [151]. The liposome could have nonometric measures providing a positive characteristic to be used in various branches of science. With such tiny measures, nanotechnology allows the introduction of drugs directly to where they are needed in the human body, minimizing side effects, adverse reactions and inadequate dosages, in addition to acting directly in the sick cell. Because they can have a nanometric size (about 100 nanometers) and a similar traits with phospholipid bilayers of the cell membrane this molecule constitutes excellent forms to be use in pharmaceutical industry, as there are possibilities of controlled drug release related to its structural flexibility in matters of size, composition, lipid bilayer fluidity and efficacy in absorbing both hydrophilic and lipophilic compounds [152].

The application of liposomes as a therapy for control of MRSA infection was demonstrated by the improvement of antimicrobial agents stability and prolonged time of action. Studies demonstrated that liposomes are being a promising formulation for antimicrobial bacteria-directed delivery and for stimulation of immunity system during an infectious disease. In this area, several studies are being conducted with Nanoparticles (NPs) as antibacterial mediators for the treatment of infections caused by multidrug-resistant bacteria (MDR), with positive results to overcome the problems of these strains, besides assisting not only the treatment but also the diagnosis of bacterial infections.

Studies indicate that silver have effective therapeutic action against Gram-positive and Gram-negative multi drug resistant (MDR) bacteria, and when silver is staggered at nanometric sizes its antimicrobial action against microorganisms greatly increases. The silver nanoparticle (AgNPS) inhibits bacterial cell biofilms, and when associated with other antibiotics AgNPS increases the susceptibility of MDR strains to antibiotics and decrease bacterial growth in biofilms, assisting in the fight of *Acinetobacter* species [153]. A study conducted by Yang, YG (2017) [154] demonstrated the use of silver nanoparticles (AgNPS) associated to kercetin biomolecule, for the treatment of *Staphylococcus aureus* and *Pseudomonas aeruginosa* isolated from milk produced by mastitis-infected goats. In this study, the researchers describe that the minimum inhibitory concentrations of AgNPS against *S.*

aureus and *P. aeruginosa* were 1 and 2 µg/ml, respectively and the AgNPS bacterial activity was related to the generation of reactive oxygen species (ROS), malondialdehyde (MDA) and the extravasation of proteins and cellular sugars. The researchers also report that the bacteria treated with AgNP had a lower lactate dehydrogenase (LDH) and low rates of adenosine triphosphate (ATP), compared with the control group. They also observed that the bacteria treated with AgNP had the deregulated expression of glutathione (GSH), and positive regulation of glutathione S-transferase (GST). In addition, the samples were negative for superoxide dismutase (SOD) and catalase (CAT), concluding that AgNP, can induce bacterial cell death because they cause physiological and biochemical alteration after bacteria treatment. This was the first study, that demonstrated the AgNPs action against MDR pathogens isolated from the milk of goats infected with subclinical mastitis [154].

The gold nanoparticle is a stable, non-toxic and biocompatible alternative, naturally synthesized in various morphologies such as nanospheres, nanorods, nanoshells and nanocrystals. They demonstrate biocompatibility, not only for cancer diagnoses and treatment, but also to inhibit and discontinue MDR biofilm. These particles are considered safe to carry therapeutic charges, such as antibiotics, active carbovalent bonding, electrostatic infiltration and encapsulation in covalent interactions [153]. The study conducted by Mocan, et al. (2016), which used gold nanoparticles (GNP) by wet chemistry, through biofunctionalization with immunoglobulin G (IgG) molecules, describe that the bacteria growth was controlled after the administration of IgG-GNPs to MRSA cultures at different concentrations and incubation periods together with laser irradiation. The results demonstrated that Biomolecule of IgG-GNPs administration associated with prolonged irradiation with laser, caused selective and prolonged bacterial death [155]. The authors suggest that GNPs can be clopped with several antibodies that target specific molecule characteristics of the bacterial membrane. Once the bacterial site is hit, the nanoparticles can be activated under infrared irradiation (NIR), modifying the energy of photons at heat, causing the rupture of bacteria cell membrane.

Niemirowicz et al. (2016) also described in his research the method of bacterial membrane rupture through magnetic nucleus nanoparticles. This method combined nanomaterials and antibiotics for bacterial therapy by MRSA membrane rupture. This research was carried out by analyzing the bactericidal activity of the human antibacterial peptide cathelicidin LL-37, synthetic ceragenins CSA-13 and CSA-131 and antibiotics of traditional use such as vancomycin and colistin, against *S. aureus* resistant to methicillin and *P. aeruginosa*. In this study, the action of nucleus-shell MNPs, isolated and in combinations with antibiotics, was evaluated by microdilution method to analyze fractional inhibitory concentration by chemiluminescence. The researchers reported that the core-wrapper magnetic nanoparticles (MNPS) act as antimicrobial agents destroying the bacterial membrane and interacting with surface proteins, in addition to nanoparticles invading biofilms destroying spore-making bacteria and being effective in combination MDR pathogens [156].

Metal nanoparticles are also being used to induce methicillin-resistant *S. aureus* cell death [157]. The use of multi-metallic nanoparticles, of bi and tri-metallic, allow better medicinal and therapeutic effectiveness to achieve a bactericidal effect like that of monometallics due to the use of lower concentrations. The joining of two metals into nanoparticles causes cell wall damage, creating a flow of cellular materials, allowing silver and gold to interact with cellular components and DNA and cause bacterial destruction. These nanoparticles can also alter cell membranes functions, such as respiration and permeability. In addition, alter sulfur proteins, phosphorus compound, as well as DNA functions [158]. A classic example is the junction of the phytogenic bimetallic nanoparticles of another and silver of the root extract of *P. zeylanica*, in the blockade of the preformed biofilm of *Acinetobacter* [153, 159].

Vancomycin is a bactericidal antibiotic widely used against infections caused by *S. aureus*, but its effectiveness does not eliminate MRSA. Yihua Pei et al. (2017) elaborated a particle based on a compound of polymers with specific functions (PpZEV), which aggregates poly (lactic acid-co-glycolic) (PLGA) as a platform for antibiotic drug delivery; with polyethylene glycol (PEG)-PLGA conjugate, to help in maintaining the polarity for drug dispensing; and finally with Eudragit E100 (dimethylaminoethyl mecrite-based copolymer) to help in encapsulating the medication together with a derivative of chitosan ZWC (Z), which stimulates the release of the pH sensitive drug. These ppZEV nanoparticles were infiltrated by macrophages due to their size of 500-1000nm thus allowing drug distribution against intracellular pathogens. The authors state that when the substance is administered intravenously its effect becomes more satisfactory because they cluster in the liver and spleen, organs affected by intracellular infection, so the PpZEV acts directly in the intracellular medium of MRSA [160].

An example of nanoparticles used as a diagnosis agent for infections caused by multidrug-resistant bacteria (MDR) is the study of Dizaji et al. (2020), which demonstrated that *Staphylococcus aureus* resistant to methicillin infection can be identified by using polymeric nanoparticles composed by Maleimide functionalized as the main carrier matrix, conjugated to a fluorescence probe of poly [9,9′-bis (6 ″ -N, N, N-trimethylammonium) hexyl) fluorene-co-alt-4,7- (2,1,3-benzothiadiazole) dibromide]. The images showed fluorescence directly to methicillin-resistant *Staphylococcus aureus* infections, in animal samples. The authors also used the nanoparticles containing vancomycin as an *in vivo* target agent that successfully controlled bacterial infection [161]. Another recent study also describes the use of nanocomplexes to eliminate multidrug-resistant bacteria and stimulate the healing of lesions in MRSA-infected diabetic patients, with the aid of laser irradiation. The researchers describe that the strategy resulted in a synergistic effect against MRSA, in which cellular integrity was affected, ATP decreased, and Glugationa (GSH) oxidized, thus accelerating the healing of MRSA-infected lesions [162].

Li Jianghua et al. (2020), carried out a work with nanoparticles (NP) made of biocompatible F-127 surfactant, tannic acid (TA) and biguanide-based poimerformin (PMET), called FTP-NPs. The authors described that FTP-NPs have bactericidal biofilm activity *in vitro* and *in vivo*, and can eliminate bacteria from inside and outside the biofilm. The results demonstrated that low concentrations (8 to 32 µg/mL) of FTP-NP can reduce in approximately 100-fold (~2 log10) MRSA cell count. This activity can be attributed to the antifouling property of the hydrophilic pole (ethylene glycol) provided by F-127. Surfactant F-127 toxicity studies demonstrated low mammalian cells toxicity *in vitro* and absence of acute toxicity after intravenous injections in mice. The authors suggest that FTP-NP may be a promising therapy for MRSA treatment [163].

In conclusion, the application of liposomes improves the stability of antimicrobial agents and extends the length of activity time, consisting in a promising formulation for bacteria targeted delivery and immune system defense. However, further research should be carried out to establish the therapeutic efficacy of nanotechnology focused on MDR, including the existing antibiotic therapies originally developed to eliminate *S. aureus* from the list of multidrug-resistant bacteria.

PHOTODYNAMIC THERAPY

Photodynamic therapy is a non-invasive form of therapy mainly used in the treatment of cancers of various types and locations and used also in the treatment of non-oncological disease as well [164]. Findings from studies suggest that PDT therapy–mechanisms and the combination of photosensitizers can be applied for the treatment of chronic inflammation been an interesting alternative in the treatment of drug-resistant bacterial infections such as MRSA [165].

The molecular mechanism of this therapy is based on three components which produce the desired effects within damaged tissues by interaction between the: photosensitizer, light with the appropriate wavelength and oxygen dissolved in the cells [166]. Currently there are two possible mechanisms for PDT, which are responsible for the antimicrobial activity of this therapy. In the first mechanism occurs the formation of reactive oxygen species (ROS) by the action of light on the photosensitizer. These radicals react with lipids and proteins leading to the reaction chain that produces oxidation [167]. In the second mechanism, the energy of the photosensitizer is transferred to molecular oxygen particles after light activation, resulting in singlet oxygen formation. Singlet oxygen can react directly with biological molecules and creates other oxygen radicals [168]. The ROS from both mechanisms reacts within the bacterial cell or nearby, inducing the bacterial death [169].

The ability of PDT to reduce the virulence of MRSA, has been associated to its effective action against *S. aureus* toxins, such as V8 protease alpha-haemolysin and sphingomyelinase, inactivating the microorganism, representing a significant advantage over conventional antibiotic strategies [170]. Other PDT mechanisms of action identified against MRSA were the DNA break-in and disappearance of the plasmid supercoiled fraction by photosensitizers and light. Besides, photosensitizers can intercalate into double-stranded DNA and cause bacterial damage. Alterations of cytoplasmic membrane proteins, disturbance of cell-wall synthesis and the appearance of multilamellar structure in MRSA dividing cells were also mechanisms associated with the damage by ROS during PDT [33, 169, 171]. These effects were exemplified in Table 3.

The application of PDT to treat skin wounds is extensively studied. Skin wounds are serious problems in public health. Their manifestations are wide-ranging and include burns, abrasions, excisional wounds, pyogenic granulomas, reverse acne, abscesses, folliculitis, keloids and fistulas. Severity varies from patient to patient, according to individual immune system and genetic aspects, which gives these lesions specific characteristics that are important for treatment definition [169, 171, 172]. Inadequate wound handling and indiscriminate use of antibiotics may contribute to treatment failure, leading to bacterial growth and resistance [32]. In skin infections, the most common agent is *Staphylococcus aureus*, and its multiresistant strain (MRSA) is equally frequent [173]. Results concerning the therapeutic effect of PDT on wound healing demonstrated that PDT accelerated diabetic wound closure rate together with reduced hyperinflammatory response, showing an important role of PDT in controlling host inflammatory reaction [33]. Also, a recent study demonstrated a photodynamic inactivation of MRSA on porcine skin using a porphyrinic photosensitizer [174]. The development of new and effective treatment therapies is important for the rapid resolution of infections, the reduction of suffering, mortality and undesirable side effects. Photodynamic therapy (PDT) could be a promising approach to improve this public health problem [32]. Table 5 indicate the recent examples of PDT to control MRSA.

Table 5. Recent examples of PDT to control MRSA

Photosensitizers	Light	Effect	Reference
[2-((4-pyridinyl)methyl)-1 Hphenalen-1-one chloride] (SAPYR)	Visible light	*In vitro* and *in vivo* Decrease in colony-forming units (CFU)	Schreine et al. 2018 [175]
Porphyrin	Light emitting diode (LED) 655 nm	*In vitro* Decrease CFU	Tasl et al. 2018 [176]
Curcumin	Light emitting diode (LED) 40mW/cm^2 8-29 J/cm^2	*In vitro* Increase in reactive oxygen species (ROS) Decrease CFU and Adhesion	Freitas et al. 2019 [171]
5-aminolevulinic acid (ALA)	LED 384J/cm^2	*In vitro* DNA and proteins damage, morphological alterations	Huang et al. 2019 [33]
Riboflavin	LED blue light 450nm 84J/cm^2	LED and LED riboflavin associated – CFU Decrease, keratinocytes cytotoxicity.	Makdoum, Heden and Backman 2019 [177]
Cobalto dopidzene oxide nanoparticle	Visive light	MRSA death, block eflux prompt	Igbal et al. 2019 [178]
Indocyanene green	Visive light	*In vitro* Morte do MRSA *In vivo* Necrose e morte do MRSA com oxacilina	Wong et al. 2019 [179]
Myrciaria cauliflora	LED blue light	*In vitro* Decrease CFU *In vivo* decreased infection improvement of healing	Santos 2019 [180]
ALA	LED blue light	*In vitro* Decrease bacterial viability	Walter et al. 2020 [181]

The results showed here demonstrate an efficacy of PDT for the treatment of MRSA infection including cutaneous strains of MRSA, what makes this technique a possible strategy for treating *S. aureus* skin infections. PDT can effectively inhibit MRSA by damaging cell membrane, cytoplasm, proteins and nucleic acid and virulence factors inactivation, showing an interesting alternative in the treatment of drug-resistant bacterial infections.

HOMEOPHATY

With the progression of physiology science, the organisms of living beings began to be understood as a psycho/neuro/immune/endocrine/metabolic unit and the view that each system acts independently became outdated. Thus, the health/disease binomial is studied by a multifactorial dynamic perspective [182].

Due to this new approach, the scientific community seeks to innovate in the treatment of diseases with alternative methods that include the entire individual. One of the main unconventional treatments used is homeopathic medicine, a system proposed by the German physician Samuel Hahnemann, which consists of healing the patient by means of medicines that strengthen the body in order to make it more competent in recovering the lost homeostasis. The basic principle of this form of treatment is the cure by the similar - *similia similibus curantur* - that is, the disease is treated by substances that cause, in healthy individuals, symptoms similar to those in the pathology to be treated [183].

In the "classic" homeopathy, the medicine prescription is based on all the signs and symptoms displayed or expressed by the ill individual [36]. The amount of peer-reviewed homeopathy research is small when compared to those of conventional drugs, but recent studies indicate that homeopathy medications have effects that can be distinguished from placebo [184, 185]. The manufacturing process of homeopathic drugs includes dilutions followed by successions, which is the shaking of the solvent with part of the chemical compounds ultra-diluted [34]. The lack of measurable levels of chemical compounds in homeopathic drugs leaves its effectiveness in check, but there is a need for new approaches to this elucidation. The dilution and suction performed in homeopathy lead to an overlap of the molecules of the mother tincture on the water molecules, creating intermolecular structures

[186, 187]. The organization between the water molecules and the active compounds of the mother tincture, forms specific electromagnetic fields according to the compounds present in the tincture. This field affects the direction of molecules electrons spins and presents a quantum effect on the structure [187, 188]. These electromagnetic waves can propagate from the drug to the patient [187], forming a quantum tangle that can have macroscopic effects on the living organism [188]. Although the effect of the electromagnetic waves on biological systems is already known, the study of radiation in homeopathic drugs and its effect on patients is complex [188]. Homeopathy ultra-molecular and quantum theory goes along with the studies on the behavior of water molecules in the concept of "Water Memory". All these studies seek to give light to the real functioning mechanism of homeopathic medicines and their effects on biological systems [187, 188].

Within the studies evaluating the applicability of homeopathy, the reports in infectious processes stand out. Reviews describe how homeopathy controls pathogens in animal models [189] and the use of homeopathy in the control of infections caused by parasites, bacteria and viruses [189, 190, 191]. Furthermore, its use reflected in an increase of cytokines production, such as Interleukin 1 (IL-1), interleukin 2 (IL-2) and interferon gamma (INF-γ), and also in reactive O_2 species as Nitric Oxide (NO) and Hydrogen Peroxide (H_2O_2). The cytokines profile exhibited indicate an immune modulation by the Th1 cell response [190, 36]. The use of homeopathy in these processes has the advantage of reducing the use of antibiotics and the risk of bacterial resistance [36]. Nevertheless, the cure of an infection must consider account two aspects: that of the agent and that of the host. Studies on the influence of homeopathy on the host is advanced [136, 189, 190], but the study on its activity on pathogen cultures is scarcer.

Passeti et al. 2014 [192], evaluate the *in vitro* growth of the bacterium *Streptococcus pyogenes* treated with the homeopathic remedies *Arnica montana*, *Gelsemiun sempervirens*, *Belladona*, *Mercurius solubillis* and isotherapics. The results indicate that *Belladona* and *S. pyogenes* isotherapic inhibit the growth of this bacterium *in vitro*, while *Arnica montanna* stimulates its growth. In another study, Passeti et al. 2016 [37], demonstrated that MRSA cultures incubated with *Belladona* or its isotherapic show a decrease in bacterial growth. The same microbial strain treated with homeopathy was more susceptible to Methicillin, with a significant drop in *in vitro* growth when the antibiotic was associated with homeopathy, compared to the treatment with homeopathy alone (Figure 4). In addition, it was observed a significant decrease in DNAse test inhibition zone after MRSA treatment with homeopathy (Figure 4). The study of Pannek et al. 2018 [193] evaluated the action of homeopathy medicines on *Escherichia coli* (*E. coli*) *in vitro* growth. The results of disc diffusion tests using homeopathy on *E. coli* cultures did not show significant inhibition on bacteria growth. Comparing the studies, it is possible that the differences in cell wall structures of both groups of bacteria, gram-positive for MRSA and *S. pyogenes*, and gram-negative for *E.* coli, may exert a role in the activity of homeopathic drugs in *in vitro* bacteria cultures. Moreover, in Passeti's work, the methodology used to test the growth inhibition was the minimum inhibitory concentration (MIC) by broth dilution method and not disc diffusion. The selection of broth dilution method was because the homeopathic medicine does not kill the bacteria in culture, but significantly inhibits their growth. Therefore, there is a need to evaluate gram-negative bacteria cultures in the same method and conditions used in Passeti's studies, for further elucidations.

The results presented by Passeti indicate that the complementary use of homeopathy may improve MRSA susceptibility to the resistant antibiotic. This innovation is of great relevance in the current picture of multi-drug resistant bacteria. Additional investigations about the activity of homeopathy over MRSA should be conducted in order to clarify the mechanisms involved and how to better improve the bacteria susceptibility to antibiotics. These studies may provide a new direction in the treatment of MRSA infections, that can be less aggressive and more efficient.

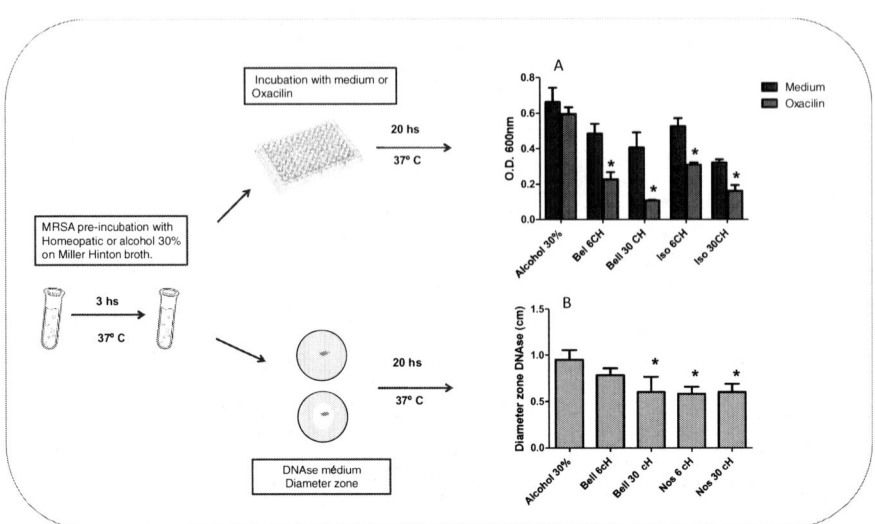

Figure 4. Action of homeopatic medicine in MRSA growth (A) and DNAse enzymatic activity (B). MRSA (0.5 Macfarland and 1/10 dilution) was pre-incubated (3 hours at 37°C) with Homeopatic or alcohol 30% on Miller Hinton broth (MH). Fifity microliters of pre-incubation suspensions were distributed in 50 μL of 4 μg/mL oxacillin solution [194] into a 96 wells microplate containing MH medium. After 20 hours at 37° C, optical density (O.D.) of bacterial growth was obtained after plate reading on a spectrophotometer at 600 nm (A). The suspensions of MRSA pre-incubation were distributed in a spot on DNAse agar medium. After incubation of 20 hours at 37°C the diameter of the DNA destruction halo was measured (B). Homeophatic were Belladona (Bell) 6CH and Bell 30CH or bacteria isotherapic (Iso) 6CH and Iso 30CH (A) or Nosode (Nos) 6CH and Nos 30CH (B). Adapted from Passeti et al. (2016) [37].

BOTANICAL MEDICINE

Plant extracts can play a central role in medicine and prevention treatment of diseases around the world. Its use was first described by Hippocrates 500 years BC, and this knowledge was immortalized by Dioscorides in the "DeMateria Medica" written 100 years BC. However, since the beginning of this century, there has been a growing interest in the study of plant species and their use in several countries. Medicinal plants and their components are among the main therapeutic resources of traditional, complementary and alternative medicine [195].

There is an interest of the scientific community in studies that prove the efficacy of plant extracts and evaluate their toxicity [196]. Currently, one of the medicine challenges that deserves special attention is the fight against multidrug-resistant bacteria. Science should be able to innovate in treatments that rewrite the future of patients with infections by multidrug-resistant bacteria such as MRSA.

Multidrug-resistant *Staphylococcus aureus* causes serious health problems in the hospital and community environment. A new strategy to deal with bacterial resistance is to explore compounds that inhibit virulence factors such as enzymes, quorum sensing, motility, surfactants and toxins, which consists a continuous field of study of anti-virulence therapy. Natural products such as catechol, quinones, manic phenolic bases and hydroxyphenyl-hydrazones show non-specific interference properties and are recognized as Pan Assay Interference Compounds (PAINS) or similar to PAINS [197]. These natural products have weak biological activities, but those are starting points for the development of new antimicrobial drugs [197].

Studies on the antimicrobial action of plant extracts has been widely explored in the scientific community [198, 199]. The results led to extracts with high antimicrobial activity and the isolation of active fractions. These studies present two methodologies, in which the extracts can be used alone or combined with antibiotics. Extracts of *Magnolia officinalis*, *Verbena officinalis*, *Momordica charantio* and *Daphne genkwa* are used with oxacillin or gentamicin to inhibit the growth of MRSA cultures. Compounds of these extracts block penicillinbindingproteins-2a proteins (PBP2a), allowing antibiotic molecules to bind to functional PBP [200].

Extracts such as *Plantanus occidentalis* and *Morinda citrifolia* have flavonoids that present antimicrobial activity against MRSA cultures [197, 201]. The most studied flavonoids are kaempferol, rhamnoside, coumarin and quercetin [197]. Hossion et al. 2011 [202] has shown that quercetin inhibits DNA gyrase and topoisomerase IV and interferes in the duplication of bacterial DNA. Other compounds studied for their action on MRSA cultures are the essential oils. Plants such as *Chamaecyparis obtusa* and Cinnamon bark present cardamom in their extract, an essential oil with an important antimicrobial action [203]. Cardamom acts on the MRSA cell membrane by increasing permeability and facilitating antibiotic penetration into the bacteria [204]. The essential oils lack of solubility problem can be solved by the formation of nanoemulsion, that increases the solubility of oils and enable their use [205]. MRSA-infected wounds have a complicating factor, the biofilm formation, which protects the bacteria from antibiotics action and facilitates the infection persistence [206]. The extracts of *Myrtis communis*, *Turnea diffusa* and *Ammopsis california* inhibit the production of lipase, hemolysin and staphyloxanthin by MRSA cultures. These extracts lead to a decrease in the biofilm formation and enhances the action of antibiotics and bacteria eradication [207]. The concomitant use of extracts with biofilm inhibition properties improves the action of antibiotics against MRSA by 95% [207].

The study of plant extracts with antimicrobial activity allows the identification of active molecules and their mechanism of action, which increases the likelihood of new antimicrobial drugs development or their use in association with known antibiotics to enhance antimicrobial activity.

CONCLUSION

Recently, WHO has been stimulating research on the development of complementary and alternative therapies to the use of antimicrobials as one of the strategies to fight antibiotics resistance. This review provides a broad overview of new and potential therapies to the treatment and prevention of MRSA infections.

The CAM mechanisms of action presented in this chapter do not aim exclusively to target the pathogen, but also to search for the rebalancing of homeostasis of the host's different organs and systems. In addition, these therapies focus on less aggressive ways of delivering available active drugs. However, the applications of these CAMs in clinical practice for the treatment of MRSA are still limited. Many studies have been carried out and it is believed that, in a near future, these therapies will broadly complement the antibiotic treatments currently in use.

Finally, due to the present restrictions in conventional antimicrobial treatments, it can be concluded that there are several promising CAM therapies towards MRSA that may be successfully used in combination with the available antibiotics, but any that could completely replace antibiotics as treatment agents.

REFERENCES

[1]   WHO - World Health Organization. 2013. *Who traditional medicine strategy: 2014-2023.* Accessed 18 Apr 2020. https://www.who.int/medicines/publications/traditional/trm_strategy14_23/en/.

[2]   Veziari, Yasamin; Kumar, Saravana and Leach, Matthew. 2018. "The development of a survey instrument to measure the barriers to the conduct and application of research in complementary and alternative medicine: a Delphi study." *BMC Complementary and Alternative Medicine.* 18:2-13.

[3]   Frass, Michael; Strassl, Robert P.; Friehs, Helmut; Müllner, Michael; Kundi, Michael and Kaye, Alan D. 2012. "Use and Acceptance of Complementary and Alternative Medicine among the General Population and Medical Personnel: A Systematic Review." *The Ochsner Journal.* 12:45–56.

[4]   MacKay, Douglas. 2003. "Can CAM therapies help reduce antibiotic resistance?" *Alternative medicine review.* 8(1):28-42.

[5]   Ernst, Edzard. 2000. "Prevalence of use of complementary/alternative medicine: a systematic review." *Bulletin of the World Health Organization.* 78(2):252–257.

[6]   Bao, Yanju; Kong, Xiangying; Yang, Liping; Liu, Rui; Shi, Zhan; Li, Weidong; Hua, Baojin and Hou, Wei. 2014. "Complementary and Alternative Medicine for Cancer Pain: An Overview of Systematic Reviews." *Evidence-Based Complementary and Alternative Medicine.* 2014: ID: 170396. doi: 10.1155/2014/170396.

[7]   Wichantuk, Pitsanee; Diraphat, Pornphan; Utrarachkij, Fuangfa; Tangwattanachuleeporn, Marut and Hirunpetcharat, Chakrit. 2018.

"Antibacterial activity of *Rafflesiakerrii* Meijer extracts against hospital isolates of methicillin-resistant *Staphylococcus aureus* (MRSA)." *Journal of Thai Interdisciplinary Research. Interdisciplinary Research Review* 13(1):40-45.

[8] WHO - World Health Organization. 2014. "Antimicrobial resistance: global report on surveillance 2014." *World Health Organization.* https://www.who.int/antimicrobialresistance/publications/surveillancereport/en/.

[9] Cunha, Mirella A.; Assunção, Gabriela L M.; Medeiros, Iara M. and Freitas, Marise R. 2016. "Antibiotic Resistance Patterns of Urinary Tract Infections." In a Northeastern Brazilian Capital. *Rev. Inst. Med. Trop.* 58(2).https://doi.org/10.1590/S1678-9946201658002.

[10] WHO - World Health Organization. 2019. "No Time to Wait: Securing the Future from Drug-Resistant Infections - Report to the Secretary-General of the United Nations." *Interagency Coordination Group on Antimicrobial Resistance.* https://www.who.int/antimicrobial-resistance/interagency-coordinationgroup/final-report/en/.

[11] De Mol, Maarten L.; Snoeck, Nico; De Maeseneire, Sofie L. and Soetaert, Wim K. 2018. "Hidden antibiotics: Where to uncover?" *Biotechnology Advances.* 36(8):2201-2218.

[12] WHO - World Health Organization. 2019. "Global Antimicrobial Resistance Surveillance System (GLASS) report: early implementation 2017-2018." *World Health Organization.* 268 pages. ISBN 978-92-4-151506-1. https://www.who.int/glass/resources/publications/early-implementation-report-2017-2018/en/.

[13] Jevons, M. Patricia. 1961. "Celbenin-resistant Staphilococci." *British Medical Journal* 1:124–125.

[14] Marshall, Caroline, Wesselingh S., McDonald M., Spelman D. 2004. "Control of endemic MRSA—what is the evidence? A personal view." *Journal Hospital Infection* 56:253–68.

[15] O'Neill, Jim. 2016. "Tackling drug-resistant infections globally: Final report and recommendations." *Review on Antimicrobial Resistance.*

Wellcome Trust and HM Government. https://amrreview.org/sites/default/files/160525_Final%20paper_with%20cover.pdf.
[16] CDC. 2019. "Antibiotic Resistance Threats in the United States, 2019." Atlanta, GA: U.S. *Department of Health and Human Services, CDC*; 2019-508 pages. doi: http://dx.doi.org/10.15620/cdc:82532.
[17] Routray, Samapika; Rath, Shakti and Mohanty, Neeta. 2019. "Prevalence of methicillin resistant *Staphylococcus aureus* isolated from saliva samples of patients with oral squamous cell carcinoma." *Journal of Oral Research*. 8(1). http://revistasacademicas.udec.cl/index.php/journal_of_oral_research/article/view/1630.
[18] Lee, Andie S.; Lencastre, Hermínia de; Garau, Javier; Kluytmans, Jan; Malhotra-Kumar, Surbhi; Peschel, Andreas and Harbarth, Stephan. 2018. Methicillin-reisitant *Staphylococcus aureus*. *Nature Reviews* 4:1-23. Article number: 18033 doi:10.1038/nrdp.2018.33.
[19] Kane, Trevor L.; Carothers, Katelyn E. and Lee, Shaun W. 2018. "Virulence Factor Targeting of the Bacterial Pathogen *Staphylococcus aureus* for Vaccine and Therapeutics." *CurrDrug Targets*. 19 (2), 111-127. doi: 10.2174/1389450117666161128123536.
[20] Acosta, Atzel C.; Costa, Mateus M.; Pinheiro Junior, José W. and Mota, Rinaldo A. 2017. "*Staphylococcus aureus* virulence factors." Medicina Veterinária (UFRPE). 11(4): 252-269.
[21] Yeaman, Michael R.; Filler, Scott G.; Chaili, Siyang; Barr, Kevin; Wang, Huiyuan; Kupferwasser, Deborah; Hennessey Jr., John P.; Fu, Yue; Schmidt, Clint S.; Edwards Jr., John E.; Xiong, Yan Q. and Ibrahim, Ashraf S. 2014. "Mechanisms of NDV-3 vaccine efficacy in MRSA skinversus invasive infection." *Proceedings of the National Academy of Sciences of the United States of America*. 111(51): 5555-5563.
[22] Haghighat, Setareh; Siadat, Seyed D.; RezayatSorkhabadi, Seyed M.; AkhavanSepahi, Abbas; Sadat, Seyed M.; Yazdi, Mohammad H. and Mahdavi, Mehdi. 2017. "Recombinant PBP2a as a vaccine candidate

against methicillin-resistant *Staphylococcus aureus*: Immunogenicity and protectivity." *Microbial Pathogenesis*. 108: 32-39.

[23] Haghighat, Setareh; Siadat, Seyed D.; Sorkhabadi, Seyed M. R.; Sepahi, Abbas Abul, and Mahdavi, Mehdi. 2017. "A novel recombinant vaccine candidate comprising PBP2a and autolysin against Methicillin Resistant *Staphylococcus aureus* confers protection in the experimental mice." *Molecular Immunology*. 91: 1-7.

[24] Majelan, Peyman A.; Mahdavi, Mehdi; Yazdi, Mohammad H.; Salimi, Elaheh and Pourmand, Mohammad R. 2019. "Recombinant Staphylococcal Antigen-F (r-ScaF), a novel vaccine candidate against methicillin resistant *Staphylococcus aureus* infection: Potency and efficacy studies." *Microbial Pathogenesis*, 127, 159–165.

[25] Saraiva, Felipe B.; Araújo, Ana C. C.; Araújo, Anna E. V. and Senna, José P. M. 2019. "Monoclonal antibody anti-PBP2a protects mice against MRSA (methicillin-resistant *Staphylococcus aureus*) infections." *Plos One*. 14(11): 1-13.

[26] Tkhilaishvili, Tamta; Wang, Lei; Tavanti, Arianna; Trampuz, Andrej and Di Luca, Mariagrazia. 2020. "Antibacterial Efficacy of Two Commercially Available Bacteriophage Formulations, Staphylococcal Bacteriophage and PYO Bacteriophage, Against Methicillin-Resistant *Staphylococcus aureus*: Prevention and Eradication of Biofilm Formation and Control of a Systemic Infection of *Galleria mellonella* Larvae." *Front. Microbiol*. 11(110): 1-15.

[27] Guo, Yunlei; Song, Guanghui; Sun, Meiling; Wang, Juan and Wang, Yi. 2020. "Prevalence and Therapies of Antibiotic-Resistance in *Staphylococcus aureus*." *Front. Cell. Infect. Microbiol*. 10(107): 1-11.

[28] Rukavina, Zora; ŠegvićKlarić, Maja; Filipović-Grčić, Jelena; Lovrić, Jasmina and Vanić, Željka. 2018. "Azithromycin-loaded liposomes for enhanced topical treatment of methicillin-resistant *Staphyloccocus aureus* (MRSA) infections." *International Journal of Pharmaceutics*. 553: 109-119.

[29] Wolfmeier, Heidi; Mansour, Sarah C.; Liu, Leo T.; Pletzer, Daniel; Draeger, Annette; Babiychuk, Eduard B. and Hancock, Robert E. W. 2018. "Liposomal Therapy Attenuates Dermonecrosis Induced by Community-Associated Methicillin-Resistant *Staphylococcus aureus* by Targeting α-Type Phenol-Soluble Modulins and α-Hemolysin." *EBioMedicine*. 33, 211-217.

[30] Scriboni, Andreia B.; Couto, Verônica M.; Ribeiro, Lígia N. M.; Freires, Irlan A.; Groppo, Francisco C.; de Paula, Eneida; Franz-Montan, Michelle andCogo-Müller, Karina. 2019. Fusogenic Liposomes Increase the Antimicrobial Activity of Vancomycin Against *Staphylococcus aureus* Biofilm. *Front. Pharmacol*. 10:1401. doi: 10.3389/fphar.2019.01401.

[31] Briggs, Timothy; Blunn, Gordon; Hislop, Simon; Ramalhete, Rita; Bagley, Caroline; McKenna, David; and Coathup, Melanie. 2018. "Antimicrobial photodynamic therapy—a promising treatment for prosthetic joint infections." *Lasers in Medical Science*. 33: 523-532.

[32] Oyama, Jully; Ramos-Milaré, Ana C. F. H.; Lera-Nonose, Daniele S. S. L.; Nesi-Reis, Vanessa; Demarchi, Izabel G.; Aristides, Sandra M. A.; Teixeira, Jorge J. V.; Silveira, Thaís G. V. andLonardoni, Maria Valdrinez C. 2020. "Photodynamic therapy in wound healing in vivo: a systematic review." *Photodiagnosis and Photodynamic Therapy*. doi: 10.1016/j.pdpdt.2020.101682.

[33] Huang, Jianhua; Guo, Mingquan; Jin, Shengkai; Wu, Minfeng; Yang, Chen; Zhang, Guolong; Wang, Peiru; Ji, Jie; Zeng, Qingyu; Wang, Xiuli and Wang, Hongwei. 2019. "Antibacterial Photodynamic Therapy Mediated by 5-aminolevulinic acid on *methicillin-resistant Staphylococcus aureus*." *Photodiagnosis and Photodynamic Therapy*. doi: https://doi.org/10.1016/j.pdpdt.2019.09.008.

[34] *Farmacopéia Homeopática Brasileira*. 3rd edn. Brazil: Agência Nacional de Vigilância Sanitária (ANVISA). Available at: http://www.anvisa.gov.br/hotsite/farmacopeiabrasileira/conteudo/3a_2011. [*Brazilian Homeopathic Pharmacopoeia*]

[35] Fontaine, Pierre and Lawson, Karen. 2009. "Classical Homeopathy Approach in the Treatment of Methicillin-Resistant *Staphylococcus*

aureus." *Explore: The Journal of Science and Healing.* 5 (6): 347-351.

[36] Fixsen, Alison. 2018. "Homeopathy in the Age of Antimicrobial Resistance: Is It a Viable Treatment for Upper Respiratory Tract Infections?" *Homeopathy*, 107 (02): 99-114.

[37] Passeti, Tânia A.; Bissoli, Leandro R.; Macedo, Ana P.; Libame, Registila B.; Diniz, Susana N. andWaisse, Silvia. 2016. "Action of antibiotic oxacillin on in vitro growth of *methicillin-resistant Staphylococcus aureus* (MRSA) previously treated with homeopathic medicines." *Homeopathy*. 106 (1), 27-31.

[38] Abul, Abbas K.; Lichtman, Andrew H. and Pillai, Shiv. 2017. "B cell activiation and antibody production." In *Cellular and Molecular Immunology*. Edited by Elsevier. 9th Edition ISBN: 9780323479783, eBook ISBN: 9780323523226. Pg. 608.

[39] Köhler, Giessen and Milstein, César. 1975. Continuous cultures of fused cells secreting antibody of predefined specificity. Nature 256: 495 – 497.

[40] Yokoyama, W. 1995. "Production of monoclonal antibodies: induction of immune responses." p. 2.5.4-2.5.8. In J. E. Coligan, A. M. Kruisbeek, D. H. Margulies, E. M. Shevach, and W. Strober (ed.), *Current protocols in immunology*, 71(12): 6864–6870.

[41] Rouha, Harald; Badarau, Adriana; Visram,; Battles, Michael B.; Prinz, Bianka; Magyarics, Zoltán; Nagy, Gábor; Mirkina, Irina; Stulik, Lukas; Zerbs, Manuel; Jägerhofer, Michaela; Maierhofer, Barbara; Teubenbacher, Astrid; Dolezilkova, Ivana; Gross, Karin; Banerjee, Srijib; Zauner, Gerhild; Malafa, Stefan; Zmajkovic, Jakub; Maier, Sabine; Mabry, Robert; Krauland, Eric; Wittrup, Dane K.; Gerngross, Tillman U. and Nagy, Eszter. 2015. "Five birds, one stone: neutralization of alpha-hemolysin and 4 bi-component leukocidins of *Staphylococcus aureus* with a single human monoclonal antibody." *MAbs.* 7(1):243–254.

[42] Sause, William E.; Buckley, Peter T.; Strohl, William R.; Lynch, Anthony S.; and Torres, Victor J. 2016 "Antibody-Based Biologics

and Their Promise to Combat *Staphylococcus aureus* Infections." *Trends Pharmacol Sci.* 37(3):231-24.

[43] Jing, Chendi; Liu, Chenghua; Liu, Fangjie; Gao, Yaping; Liu, Yu; Guan, Zhangchun; Xuan, Bo; Yu, Yanyan and Yang, Guang. 2018. "Novel human monoclonal antibodies targeting the F subunit of leukocidins reduce disease progression and mortality caused by *Staphylococcus aureus.*" *BMC Microbiol.* 18(181): 1-10. https://doi.org/10.1186/s12866-018-1312-7.

[44] Liu, Yuanyuan; Song, Zhen; Ge, Shuang; Zhang, Jinyong; Xu, Limin; Yang, Feng; Lu, Dongshui; Luo, Ping; Gu, Jiang; Zou, Quanming and Zeng, Hao. 2020. "Determining the immunological characteristics of a novel human monoclonal antibody developed against staphylococcal enterotoxin B." *Hum Vaccin Immunother.* 10:1-11.

[45] Hua, Lia; Cohen, Taylor S.; Shi, Yan; Datta, Vikram; Hilliard, Jamese J.; Tkaczyk, Christine; Suzich, Joann; Stover, Kendall C. and Sellman, Bret R. 2015. "MEDI4893* promotes survival and extends the antibiotic treatment window in a *Staphylococcus aureus* immunocompromised pneumonia model." *Antimicrob Agents Chemother.* 59:4526–4532.

[46] Yu, Xiang-Qing; Robbie, Gabriel J.; Wu, Yuling; Esser, Mark T.; Jensen, Kathryn; Schwartz, Howard I.; Bellamy, Terramika; Hernandez-Illas, Martha and Jafri, Hasan S. 2016. "Safety, tolerability, and pharmacokinetics of MEDI4893, an investigational, extended-half-life, anti-*Staphylococcus aureus* alpha-toxin human monoclonal antibody, in healthy adults." *Antimicrob Agents Chemother.* 61(1): e01020–16. doi: 10.1128/AAC.01020-16.

[47] François, Bruno; Mercier, Emmanuelle; Gonzalez, Céline; Asehnoune, Karim; Nseir, Saad; Fiancette, Maud; Desachy, Arnaud; Plantefève, Gaëtan; Meziani, Ferhat; Lame, Paul-André and Laterre, Pierre-François. 2018. "Safety and tolerability of a single administration of AR-301, a human monoclonal antibody, in ICU patients with severe pneumonia caused by *Staphylococcus aureus*: first-in-human trial." *Intensive Care Med.* 44:1787–1796.

[48] Burnie, James P.; Matthews, Ruth C.; Carter, Tracey; Beaulieu, Elaine; Donohoe, Michael; Chapman, Caroline; Williamson, Peter; and Hodgetts, Samantha J. 2000. "Identification of an immunodominant ABC transporter in *methicillin-resistant Staphylococcus aureus* infections." *Infect Immun.* 68(6):3200–3209.

[49] Otto, Michael. 2010. "Novel targeted immunotherapy approaches for staphylococcal infection." *Expert opinion on biological therapy.* 10(7):1049–1059.

[50] Baker, Monya. 2006. "Anti-infective antibodies: finding the path forward." *Nat Biotechnol.* 24(12):1491–1493.

[51] Hall, Andrea E.; Domanski, Paul J.; Patel, Pratiksha R.; Vernachio, John H.; Syribeys, Peter J.; Gorovits, Elena L.; Johnson, Michael A.; Ross, Julia M.; Hutchins, Jeff T. and Patti, Joseph M. 2003 "Characterization of a protective monoclonal antibody recognizing *Staphylococcus aureus* MSCRAMM protein clumping factor A." *Infect Immun.* 71(12):6864-70.

[52] Patti. Joseph M. 2004 "A humanized monoclonal antibody targeting *Staphylococcus aureus*." *Vaccine.* 22: 39-43.

[53] Weems Jr., John J.; Steinberg, James P.; Filler, Scott; Baddley, John W.; Corey, Ralph G.; Sampathkumar, Priya; Winston, Lisa; John, Joseph F.; Kubin, Christine J.; Talwani, Rohit; Moore, Thomas; Patti, Joseph M.; Hetherington, Seth; Texter, Michele; Wenzel, Eric;. Kelley, Violet A. and Fowler Jr., Vance G. 2006. "Phase II, randomized, double-blind, multicenter study comparing the safety and pharmacokinetics of tefibazumab to placebo for treatment of *Staphylococcus aureus* bacteremia." *Antimicrob Agents Chemother.* 50(8):2751–2755.

[54] John Jr., Joseph F. 2006. "Drug evaluation: tefibazumab--a monoclonal antibody against staphylococcal infection." *Current opinion in molecular therapeutics.* 8(5):455–460.

[55] Dejonge, Mitchell; Burchfield, David; Bloom, Barry; Duenas, Maria; Walker, Whit; Polak, Mark; Jung, Elizabeth; Millard, Dietra; Schelonka, Robert; Eyal, Fabien; Morris, Amy; Kapik, Barry; Roberson, Destrey; Kesler, Karen; Patti, Joe and Hetherington, Seth.

2007. "Clinical trial of safety and efficacy of INH-A21 for the prevention of nosocomial staphylococcal bloodstream infection in premature infants." *J Pediatr.* 151(3):260-5.

[56] *Safety and Efficacy of Veronate® Versus Placebo in Preventing Nosocomial Staphylococcal Sepsis in Premature Infants* [Internet]. 2005. Available from: https://clinicaltrials.gov/ct2/show/NCT00 113191.

[57] *Aurexis® in Cystic Fibrosis Subjects Chronically Colonized With Staphylococcus aureus in Their Lungs* [Internet]. 2005. Available from: https://clinicaltrials.gov/ct2/show/NCT00198289.

[58] *Clinical Trial Comparing Safety and Pharmacokinetics of Standard Antibiotic Therapy, Plus Aurexis® or Placebo, for Treatment of Staphylococcus aureus Bacteremia (SAB)* [Internet]. 2005. https://clinicaltrials.gov/ct2/show/NCT00198302.

[59] Weisman, Leonard E.; Thackray, Helen M.; Garcia-Prats, Joseph A.; Nesin, Mirjana; Schneider, Joseph H.; Fretz, Jennifer; Kokai-Kun, John F.; Mond, James J.; Kramer, William G. and Fischer, Gerald W. 2009. "Phase 1/2 double-blind, placebo-controlled, dose escalation, safety, and pharmacokinetic study of pagibaximab (BSYX-A110), an antistaphylococcal monoclonal antibody for the prevention of staphylococcal bloodstream infections, in very-low-birth-weight neonates." *Antimicrobial agents and chemotherapy.* 53(7):2879–2886.

[60] *Safety and Pharmacokinetics Study in Adults for the Prevention of S. Epidermidis Infection in Low Birth Weight Infants* [Internet]. 2008. https://clinicaltrials.gov/ct2/show/NCT00636285.

[61] Weisman, Leonard E.; Thackray, Helen M.; Steinhorn, Robin H.; Walsh, William F.; Lassiter, Herbert A.; Dhanireddy, Ramasubbareddy; Brozanski, Beverly S.; Palmer, Kristine G. H.; Trautman, Michael S.; Escobedo, Marilyn; Meissner, Cody H.; Sasidharan, Pontthenkandath; Fretz, Jennifer; Kokai-Kun, John F.; Kramer, William G.; Fischer, Gerald W. and Mond, James J. 2011. "A randomized study of a monoclonal antibody (pagibaximab) to prevent staphylococcal sepsis." *Pediatrics.* 128(2):271-9.

[62] *Safety and efficacy of Pagibaximab injection in very low birth weight neonates for prevention of staphylococcal sepsis* [Internet]. 2011. Available from: https://clinicaltrials.gov/ct2/show/study/NCT00646399.

[63] *Safety, pharmacokinetics, pharmacodynamics, and clinical activity study in vlbw neonates of BSYX-A110 (N003).* [Internet]. 2008. https://clinicaltrials.gov/ct2/show/NCT00631800.

[64] *Safety and pharmacokinetics study in vlbw neonates with BSYX-A110 (N002).* [Internet]. 2008. https://clinicaltrials.gov/ct2/show/NCT00631878.

[65] *Aurograb and vancomycin in MRSA infection.* [Internet]. 2005. https://clinicaltrials.gov/ct2/show/NCT00217841.

[66] *Prevention of S. aureus pneumonia study in mechanically ventilated subjects who are heavily colonized with S. aureus.* [Internet]. 2016. https://clinicaltrials.gov/ct2/show/NCT02940626.

[67] *A phase 1 study to evaluate the safety, tolerability, and pharmacokinetics of MEDI4893 in Healthy Adult Subjects* [Internet]. 2013. https://clinicaltrials.gov/ct2/show/NCT01769417.

[68] *A phase 2 randomised, double-blind, placebo-controlled, single-dose, dose-ranging study of the efficacy and safety of medi4893, a human monoclonal antibody against Staphylococcus aureus alpha toxin in mechanically ventilated adult subjects.* [Internet]. 2014. https://clinicaltrials.gov/ct2/show/NCT02296320.

[69] *Safety, pharmacokinetics and efficacy of KBSA301 in Severe Pneumonia (S. aureus).* [Internet]. 2012. https://clinicaltrials.gov/ct2/show/NCT01589185.

[70] *Adjunctive therapy to antibiotics in the treatment of S. aureus ventilator-associated pneumonia with AR-301 (AR-301-002)* [Internet]. 2019. https://clinicaltrials.gov/ct2/show/NCT03816956.

[71] Varshney, Avanish K.; Kuzmicheva, Galina A.; Lin, Jian; Sunley, Kevin M.; Bowling Jr., Rodney A.; Kwan, TzuYu; Mays, Heather R.; Rambhadran, Anu; Zhang, Yanfeng; Martin, Rebecca L.; Cavalier, Michael C.; Simard, John and Shivaswamy, Sushma . 2018. "A natural human monoclonal antibody targeting *Staphylococcus* Protein

A protects against *Staphylococcus aureus* bacteremia." *Plos One* 13(1): e0190537. https://doi.org/10.1371/journal.pone.0190537.

[72] Huynh Elizabeth, Rajora Maneesha A, Zheng Gang . 2016. "Multimodal micro, nano, and size conversion ultrasound agents for imaging and therapy." *Wiley Interdiscip Rev Nanomed Nanobiotechnol.* 8(6):796-813.

[73] *A Study of the Safety and Efficacy of 514G3 in Subjects Hospitalized With Bacteremia Due to Staphylococcus aureus* [Internet]. 2015. https://clinicaltrials.gov/ct2/show/NCT02357966.

[74] Proctor, Richard A. 2015. "Recent development for *Staphylococcus aureus* vaccines: Clinical and basic science challenges." *European Cells and Materials* 30:315-326.

[75] Pozzi, Clarissa; Olaniyi, Reuben; Liljeroos, Lassi; Galgani, Ilaria; Rappuoli, Rino, and Bagnoli, Fabio. 2016. "Vaccines for *Staphylococcus aureus* and target populations." *Current Topics in Microbiology and Immunology* 409:491-528.

[76] Miller, Lloyd S.; Fowler Jr., Vance G.; Shukla, Sanjay K.; Rose, Warren E. and Proctor, Richard A. 2020. "Development of a vaccine against *Staphylococcus aureus* invasive infections: Evidence based on human immunity, genetics and bacterial evasion mechanisms." *FEMS Microbiology Reviews* 44:123-153.

[77] Botelho-Nevers, Elisabeth; Verhoeven, Paul; Paul, Stephane; Grattard, Florence; Pozzetto, Bruno; Berthelot, Philippe and Lucht, Frederic. 2013. "Staphylococcal vaccine development: review of past failures and plea for future evaluation of vaccine efficacy not only on staphylococcal infections but also on mucosal carriage." *Expert Reviews of Vaccines* 12(11):1249-1259.

[78] Daum, Robert S. and Spellberg, Brad. 2012. "Progress toward a *Staphylococcus aureus* vaccine." *Vaccines* 54:560-567.

[79] Proctor, Richard A. 2012. "Is there a future for a *Staphylococcus aureus* vaccine?" *Vaccine* 30:2921-2927.

[80] Fowler Jr., Vance G. and Proctor, Rihcard A. 2014. "Where does a *Staphylococcus aureus* vaccine stand?" *Clinical Microbiology and Infection* 20(Suppl. 5):66-75.

[81] Giersing, Birgitte K.; Dastgheyb, Sana S.; Modjarrad, Kayvon; Moorthy, Vasse. 2016. "Status of vaccine research and development of vaccines for *Staphylococcus aureus.*" 34:2962-2966.

[82] Mohamed, Naglaa; Wang, Mian Ying; Le Huec, Jean-Charles; Liljenqvist, Ulf; Scully, Ingrid L.; Baber, James; Begier, Elizabeth; Jansen, Kathrin U.; Gurtman, Alejandra and Anderson, Annaliesa S. 2017. "Vaccine development to prevent *Staphylococcus aureus* surgical-site infections." *BJS Society* 104:e-41-e54. doi: 10.1002/bjs.10454.

[83] Proctor, Richard A. 2019. "Immunity t *Staphylococcus aureus*: Implications for vaccine development." *Microbiology Spectrum* 7(4):GPP3-0037-2018. doi:10.1128/microbiolspec.GPP3-0037-2018.

[84] Bagnoli, Fabio; Bertholet, Sylvie and Grandi, Guido. 2012. "Inferring reasons for the failure of *Staphylococcus aureus* vaccines in clinical trials." *Frontiers in Cellular and Infection Microbiology* 2(16):1-4. doi: https://doi.org/10.3389/fcimb.2012.00016.

[85] Von Eiff, Christof. 2008. "*Staphylococcus aureus* small colony variants: a challenge to microbiologists and clinicians." *International Journal of Antimicrobial Agents* 31: 507-510.

[86] Harro, Janette M.; Peters, Brian M.; O'May, Graeme A.; Archer, Nathan; Kerns, Patrick; Prabhakara, Ranjani and Shirtliff, Mark E. 2010. "Vaccine development in *Staphylococcus aureus:* taking the biofilm phenotype into consideration." *FEMS Immunology and Medical Microbiology* 59:306-323.

[87] Cheng, Alice G.; McAdow, Molly; Kim, Hwan K.; Bae, Taeko; Missiakas, Dominique M. and Schneewind, Olaf. 2010. "Contribution of coagulase towards *Staphylococcus aureus* disease and protective immunity." *Plos Pathogens* 6(8):e1001036. doi: 10.1371/journal.ppat.1001036.

[88] Kobayashi, Scott D.; Malachowa, Natalia and DeLeo, Frank R. 2015. "Pathogenesis of *Staphylococcus aureus* abscesses." *The American Journal of Pathology* 185:1518-1527.

[89] Raffat, Dina; Otto, Michael; Reppschläger, Kevin; Iqbal, Jawad and Holtfreter, Silva. 2019. "Fighting *Staphylococcus aureus* biofilms with monoclonal antibodies." *Trends Microbiology* 27(4):303-322.

[90] Löffler, Bettina; Hussain, Muzzaffar; Grundmeier, Mathias; Brück, Michaela; Holzing, Dirk; Varga, Georg; Roth, Johannes; Kahl, Barbara C.; Proctor, Richard A. and Peters Georg. 2010. "*Staphylococcus aureus* Panton-Valentine Leukocidin is a very potent cytotoxic factor for human neutrophils." *PloS Pathogens* 6(1):e1000715. doi:10.1371/journal.ppat.1000715.

[91] Salgado-Pabón, Wilmara and Schlievert, Patrick M. 2014. "Models matter: the search for an effective *Staphylococcus aureus* vaccine." *Nature Review Microbiology* 1-7. doi:10.1038/nrmicro3308.

[92] Fattom, Ali; Matalom, Albert; Buerkert, John; Taylor, Kimverly; Damaso, Silvia and Boutriau, Dominique. 2015. "Efficacy profile of bivalent *Staphylococcus aureus* glycoconjugated vaccine in adults on hemodialysis: Phase III randomized study." *Human Vaccines and Immunotherapeutics* 11(3):632-641.

[93] McNeely, Tessie B.; Shah, Najaf A.; Fridman, Arthur; Joshi, Amita; Hartzel, Jonathan S.; Keshari, Ravi S.; Lupu, Florea and DiNubile, Mark J. 2014. "Mortality among recipients of the Merck V710 *Staphylococcus aureus* vaccine after postoperative *S. aureus* infections: An analysis of possible contributing host factors." *Human Vaccine & Immunotherapeutics* 10(12):3513-3516.

[94] Irene, Carmela; Fantappiè, Laura; Caproni, Elena; Zerbini, Francesca; Anesi, Andrea; Tomasi, Michele; Zanella, Ilaria; Stupia, Simone; Prete, Stefano; Valensin, Silvia; König, Enrico; Frattini, Luca; Gagliardi, Assunta; Isaac, Smine J.; Grandi, Alberto; Guella, Graziano and Grandi, Guido. 2019. "Bacterial outer membrane vesicles engineered with lipidated antigens as a platform for *Staphylococcus aureus* vaccine." *PNAS* 116(43):21780-21788.

[95] Cheng, Brian L.; Nielsen; Travis B.; Pantapalangkoor, Paul; Zhao, Fan; Lee, Jean C.; Montgomery, Christopher P.; Luna, Brian; Spellberg, Brad and Daum, Robert S. 2017. "Evaluation of serotypes 5 and 8 capsular polysaccharides inprotection against *Staphylococcus*

aureus in murine models of infection." *Human Vaccines & Immunotherapeutics* 13: 1609-1614.

[96] Adhikari, Rajan P.; Karauzum, Hatice; Sarwar, Jawad; Abaandou, Laura; Mahmoudieh, Mahta; Boroun, Atefeh R.; Vu, Hong; Nguyen, Tam; Devi, Sathya; Shulenin, Sergey; Warfield, Kelly L. and Aman, Javad M. 2012. "Novel structurally designed vaccine for *S. aureus* α-hemolysin: protection against bacteremia and pneumonia." *PloS One*. 7(6): e38567. doi: 10.1371/journal.pone.0038567.

[97] Moscoso, Miriam; García, Patricia; Cabral, Maria P.; Rumbo, Carlos andBou, Germán. 2018. "A D-Alanine Auxotrophic Live vaccine is effective against lethal infection caused by *Staphylococcus aureus*." *Virulence* 9(1):604-620.

[98] Liuyang Yang, Heng Zhou, Ping Cheng, Yun Yang, Yanan Tong, QianfeiZuo, Qiang Feng, Quanming Zou, Hao Zeng2018. A novel bivalent fusion vaccine induces broad immunoprotection against *Staphylococcus aureus* infection in different murine models. *Clin Immunol.* 188:85-93.

[99] Levy, Jack; Licini, Laurent; Haelterman, Edwige; Moris, Philippe; Lestrate, Pascal; Damaso, Silvia; Van Belle, Pascale and Boutriau, Dominique. 2015. "Safety and Immunogenicity of an Investigational 4-component *Staphylococcus aureus* vaccine with or without AS03B adjuvant: Results of a Randomized Phase I Trial." *Human Vaccines & Immunotherapeutics.* 11(3):620-631.

[100] Torre, Antonina; Bacconi, Marta; Sammicheli, Chiara; Galletti, Bruno; Laera, Donatello; Fontana, Maria R.; Grandi, Guido; De Gregorio, Ennio; Bagnoli, Fabio; Nuti, Sandra; Bertholet, Sylvie and Bensi Giuliano. 2015. "Four-component *Staphylococcus aureus* vaccine 4C-staph enhances Fc _ receptor expression in neutrophils and monocytes and mitigates *S. aureus* infection in neutropenic mice." *Infection and Immunity* 83(8):3157–63.

[101] Mancini, Francesca; Monaci, Elisabetta; Lofano, Giuseppe; Torre, Antonina; Bacconi, Marta; Tavarini, Simona; Sammicheli, Chiara; Arcidiacono, Letizia; Galletti, Bruno; Laera, Donatello; Pallaoro, Michele; Tuscano, Giovanna; Fontana, Maria R.; Bensi, Giuliano;

Grandi, Guido; Rossi-Paccani, Silvia; Nuti, Sandra; Rappuoli, Rino; De Gregorio, Ennio; Bagnoli, Fabio; Soldaini, Elisabetta and Bertholet, Sylvie. 2016. "One Dose of *Staphylococcus aureus* 4C-Staph Vaccine Formulated with a Novel TLR7-Dependent Adjuvant Rapidly Protects Mice through Antibodies, Effector CD4+ T Cells, and IL-17A." *PLoS ONE* 11(1): e0147767. doi:10.1371/journal.pone.0147767.

[102] Schmidt, Clint S.; White, Christopher J.; Ibrahim, Ashraf S.; Filler, Scott G.; Fu, Yue; Yeaman, Michael R.; Edwards Jr, John E. and Hennessey Jr., John P. 2012. "NDV-3, a recombinant alum-adjuvanted vaccine for Candida and *Staphylococcus aureus*, is safe and immunogenic in healthy adults." *Vaccine* 30:7594-600.

[103] Roetzer, Andreas; Jilma, Bernd and Eibl, Martha M. 2017. "Vaccine against toxic shock syndrome in a first-in-man clinical trial." *Expert Rev Vaccines.* 16, 81-3.

[104] Chen, Wilbur H.; Pasetti, Marcela F.; Adhikari, Rajan P.; Baughman, Holly; Douglas, Robin; El-Khorazaty, Jill; Greenberg, Nancy; Holtsberg, Frederick W.; Liao, Grant C.; Reymann, Mardi K.; Wang, Xiaolin; Warfield, Kelly L. and Aman, M Javad. 2016. "Safety and immunogenicity of a parenterally administered, structure-based rationally modified recombinant staphylococcal enterotoxin B protein vaccine, STEBVax." *Clinical and Vaccine Immunology.* 23, 918-925.

[105] Landrum, Michael L.; Lalani, Tahaniyat; Niknian, Minoo; Maguire, Jason D.; Hospenthal, Duane R.; Fattom, Ali; Taylor, Kimberly; Fraser, Jamie; Wilkins, Kenneth; Ellis, Michael W.; Kessler, Paul D.; Fahim, Rafaat E. F. and Tribble, David R. 2017. "Safety and immunogenicity of a recombinant *Staphylococcus aureus* α-toxoid and a recombinant Panton-Valentine leukocidin subunit, in healthy adults." *Human Vaccines & Immunotherapeutics* 13:791-801.

[106] Anderson, Annaliesa S.; Miller, Alita A.; Donald, Robert G. K.; Scully, Ingrid L.; Nanra, Jasdeep S.; Cooper, David and JansenKathrin U. 2012. "Development of a multicomponent *Staphylococcus aureus* vaccine designed to counter multiple bacterial

virulence factors." *Human Vaccines & Immunotherapeutics* 8:1585–1594.

[107] Creech, C. Buddy; Frenck Jr, Robert W.; Sheldon, Eric A.; Seiden, David J.; Kankam, Martin K.; Zito, Edward T.; Girgenti, Douglas; Severs, Joseph M.; Immermann, Frederick W.; McNeil, Lisa K.; Cooper, David; Jansen, Kathrin U.; Gruber, William; Eiden, Joseph; Anderson, Annaliesa S. and Baber, James. 2017. "Safety, tolerability, and immunogenicity of a single dose 4-antigen or 3-antigen *Staphylococcus aureus* vaccine in healthy older adults: Results of a randomized trial." *Vaccine*. 35:385-394.

[108] Begier, Elizabeth; Seiden, David J.; Patton, Michael; Zito, Edward; Severs, Joseph; Cooper, David; Eiden, Joseph; Gruber, William C.; Jansen, Kathrin U.; Anderson, Annaliesa S. and Gurtman, Alejandra. 2017. "SA4Ag, a 4-antigen *Staphylococcus aureus* vaccine, rapidly induces high levels of bacteria-killing antibodies." *Vaccine*. 35:1132-1139.

[109] Frenck Jr, Robert W.; Buddy, Creech, C.; Sheldon, Eric A.; Seiden, David J.; Kankam, Martin K.; Baber, James; Zito, Edward; Hubler, Robin; Eiden, Joseph; Severs, Joseph M.; Sebastian, Shite; Nanra, Jasdeep; Jansen, Kathrin U.; Gruber, William C.; Anderson, Annaliesa S. and Girgenti, Douglas. 2017. "Safety, tolerability, and immunogenicity of a 4-antigen *Staphylococcus aureus* vaccine (SA4Ag): results from a first-in-human randomized, placebo-controlled phase 1/2 study." *Vaccine*. 35:375-384.

[110] Gurtman, Alejandra; Begier, Elizabeth; Mohamed, Naglaa; Baber, James; Sabharwal, Charulata J.; Haupt, Richard M.; Edwardsd, Holly; Cooper, David; Jansen Kathrin U. and Anderson. Annaliesa S. 2019. "The development of a *Staphylococcus aureus* fou antigen vaccine for use prior to elective orthopedic surgery." *Human Vaccines & Immunotherapeutics* 15(2):358-370.

[111] Ferraro, Alessandra; Buonocore, Sofia M.; Auquier, Philippe; Nicolas, Isabelle; Wallemacq, Hugues; Boutriau, Dominique and Van der Most, Robert G. 2019. "Role and plasticity of Th1 and Th17

responses in immunity to *Staphylococcus aureus*." *Human Vaccines and Immunotherapeuthics* 15(12):2980-2992.

[112] Diep, Binh A.; Le, Vien T. M.; Badiou, Cedric; Le, Hoan N.; Pinheiro, Marcos G.; Duong, Au H.; Wang, Xing; Dip, Etyene C.; Aguiar-Alves, Fábio; Basuino, Li; Marbach, Helene; Mai, Thuy T.; Sarda, Marie N.; Kajikawa, Osamu; Matute-Bello, Gustavo; Tkaczyk, Christine; Rasigade, Jean-Phlippe; Sellman, Bret R.; Chambers, Henry F. and Lina, Gerald. 2016. "IVIG-mediated protection against necrotizing pneumonia caused by MRSA." *Infectious Disease* 8(357ra124):1-13. doi: 10.1126/scitranslmed.aag1153.

[113] Ansari, Shamshul; Jha, Rajesh K.; Mishra, Shyam K; Tiwari, Birendra R. and Asaad, Ahmed M. 2019. "Recent advances in *Staphylococcus aureus* infection: focus on vaccine development." *Infection and Drug Resistance* 12:1243-1255.

[114] Dupont, Christopher D.; Scully, Ingrid L.; Zimmisky, Ross M.; Monian, Brinda; Rossitto, Christina P.; OÇonnell, Ellen B.; Jansen, Kathrin U.; Andreson, Annaliesa S. and Love, J. Christopher. 2018. "Two vaccines for *Staphylococcus aureus* induce a B-cell-mediated immune response." *Therapeuthics and Prevention* 3(4): e00217-18. doi: https://doi.org/10.1128/mSphere.00217-18.

[115] Zhang, Fan; Ledue, Olivia; Jun, Maria; Goulart, Cibelly; Malley, Richard and Lu, Ying-Jie. 2018. "Protection against *Staphylococcus aureus* colonization and infection by B- and T-cell-mediated mechanisms." *Host-Microbe Biology* 9(5): e01949-18. doi: https://doi.org/10.1128/mBio.01949-18.

[116] Deng, Jian; Wang, Xiaolei; Zhang, Bao-Zhong; Gao, Peng; Lin, Qiubin; Kao, Richard Yi-Tsun; Gustafsson, Kenth; Yuen, Kwok-Yung and Huanga, Jian-Dong. 2019. "Broad and Effective Protection against *Staphylococcus aureus* is elicited by a multivalent vaccine formulated with novel Antigens." *Therapeutics and Prevention* 4(5): e00362-19. doi: https://doi.org/10.1128/mSphere.00362-19.

[117] Cruciani, Melania; Sandini, Silvia; Etna, Marilena P.; Giacomini, Elena; Camilli, Romina; Severa, Martina; Rizzo, Fabiana; Bagnoli, Fabio; Hiscott, John andCoccia, Eliana M. 2019. "Differential

Responses of Human Dendritic Cells to Live or Inactivated *Staphylococcus aureus:* Impact on Cytokine Production and T Helper Expansion." *Frontiers Immunology* 10(Article 2622):1-11. doi: 10.3389/fimmu.2019.02622.

[118] Brown, Aisling F.; Leech, John M.; Rogers, Thomas R.and McLoughlin, Rachel M. 2014. "*Staphylococcus aureus* colonization: modulation of host immune response and impact on human vaccine design." *Frontiers in Immunology* 4:1-29. Article 507. doi: 10.3389/fimmu.2013.00507 ONLINE.

[119] Si, Touhul; Zhao, Fan; Beesetty, Pavani; Weiskopf, Daniela; Li, Zhaotao; Tian, Qiaomu; Alegre, Maria-Luisa; Sette, Alessandro; Chong, Anita S. and Montgomery, Christopher P. 2020. "Inhibition of protective immunity against *Staphylococcus aureus* infection by MHC-restricted immunodominance is overcome by vaccination." *Immunology* 6:eaaw7713 pages 1-14. doi:10.1126/sciadv.aaw7713.

[120] DeLorenzo, Gerald N.; Nelson, Charlotte L.; Scott, William K.; Allen, Andrew S.; Ray, G. Thomas; Tsai, Ai-Lin; Quesenberry Jr, Charles P. and Fowler Jr, Vance G. 2017. "Polymorphisms in HLA Class II genes are associated with susceptibility to *Staphylococcus aureus* infection in a white population." *The Journal of Infectious Diseases* 213:816-823.

[121] Gualandi, Nicole; Mu, Yi; Bamberg, Wendy M.; Dumyati, Ghinwa; Harrison, Lee H.; Lesher, Lindsey; Nadle, Joelle; Petit, Sue; Ray, Susan M.; Schaffner, William, Townes, John; McDonald, Mariana and See, Isaac. 2018. "Racial disparities in invasive methicillin-resistant *Staphylococcus aureus* infections, 2005-2014." *Clinical Infectious Diseases* 67(8):1175-1181.

[122] Cyr, Derek D.; Allen, Andrew S.; Du, Guang-jian; Ruffin, Felicia; Adams, Carlton; Thaden, Joshua T.; Maskarinec, Stacey A.; Souli, Maria;Guo, Shengru; Dykxhoorn, Derek M.; Scott, William K. and Fowler Jr, Vance G. 2017. "Evaluating genetic susceptibility to *Staphylococcus aureus* bacteremia in African Americans using admixture mapping." *Genes and Immunity* 18:95-99.

[123] Redi, David; Raffaelli, Chiara S.; Rossetti, Barbara; De Luca, Andrea; Montagnani, Francesca. 2018. "*Staphylococcus aureus* vaccine preclinical and clinical development: current state of the art." *New Microbiology* 41(3):208-213.

[124] Álvarez, Andrea; Fernández, Lúcia; Gutiérrez, Diana; Iglesias, Beatriz; Rodríguez, Ana and García, Pilar. 2019. "*Methicillin-Resistant Staphylococcus aureus* in Hospitals: Latest Trends and Treatments Based on Bacteriophages." *Journal of Clinical Microbiology* 12: e01006-19. doi: 10.1128/JCM.01006-19.

[125] Peng, Chanthol; Hanawa, Tomoko; Azam, Haeruman; LeBlanc, Cierra; Ung, Porsry; Matsuda, Takeaki; Onishi, Hiroaki; Miyanaga, Kazuhiko and Tanji, Yasunori. 2019. "Silviavirus phage ϕMR003 displays a broad host range against methicillin-resistant *Staphylococcus aureus* of human origin." *Applied Microbiology and Biotechnology* 103:7751–7765.

[126] Chang, Yoonjee; Bai, Jaewoo; Lee, Ju-Hoon and Ryu, Sangryeol. 2019. "Mutation of a *Staphylococcus aureus* temperate bacteriophage to a virulent one and evaluation of its application." *Food Microbiology*. 83:523-532.

[127] Belleghem, Jonas D. Van., Dąbrowska, Krystyna., Vaneechoutte, Mario., Barr, Jeremy J., Bollyky, Paul L. 2019. "Interactions between Bacteriophage, Bacteria, and the Mammalian Immune System." *Viruses* 11(10):1-22. doi:10.3390/v11010010.

[128] Górski, Andrzej; Międzybrodzki, Ryszard; Dąbrowska, Borysowski K; Wierzbicki, Piotr; Ohams, Monika; Korczak-Kowalska, Grażyna; Olszowska-Zaremba, Natasza; Łusiak-zelachowska, Marzena; Kłak, Marlena; Jończyk, Ewa; Kaniuga, welina; Gołaś, Aneta; Purchla, Sylwia; Beata Weber, Dąbrowska; Sławomir, Letkiewicz and Wojciech, Fortuna and Krzysztof, Szufnarowski. 2012. "Phage as a modulator of immune responses: practical implications for phage therapy." *Advance Virus Research* 83:41-71.

[129] Leitner, Lorenz; Kessler, Thomas M. and Klumpp, Jochen. 2019. "Bacteriophages: a Panacea in Neuro-Urology?" *European Urology Focus* (in press). doi.org/10.1016/j.euf.2019.10.018.

[130] Hobbs, Zack and Stephen, Abedon T. 2016. "Diversity of phage infection types and associated terminology: the problem with 'Lytic or lysogenic'." *FEMS Microbiology Letters* 363:1-8.

[131] Fernández, Lucía; Gutiérrez, Diana; García, Pilar and Rodríguez, Ana. 2019. "The Perfect Bacteriophage for Therapeutic Applications—A Quick Guide." *Antibiotics* 8:126. doi:10.3390/antibiotics8030126.

[132] Drulis-Kawa, Zuzanna; Majkowska-Skrobek, Grazyna and Maciejewska, Barbara. 2015. "Bacteriophages and Phage-Derived Proteins – Application Approaches." *Current Medicinal Chemistry* 22:1757-1773.

[133] Barrera-Rivas, Claudia I.; Valle-Hurtado, Norma A; González-Lugo, Graciela M; Baizabal-Aguirre, Víctor M; Bravo-Patiño, Alejandro; Cajero-Juárez, Marcos and Valdez-Alarcón, Juan J. 2017. "Bacteriophage Therapy: An Alternative for the Treatment of *Staphylococcus aureus* Infections in Animals and Animal Models." In: Frontiers in *Staphylococcus aureus. Intech. Open*, dx.doi.org/10.5772/65761.

[134] Lehman, Susan M; Mearns, Gillian; Rankin, Deborah; Cole, Robert A; Smrekar, Frenk; Branston, Steven D and Morales, Sandra. 2019. "Design and Preclinical Development of a Phage Product for the Treatment of Antibiotic-Resistant *Staphylococcus aureus* Infections." *Viruses*. 2019 21:11(1).

[135] Sanjay, Chhibber; Tarsem, Kaur and Sandeep, Kaur. 2013. "Co-therapy using lytic bacteriophage and linezolid: effective treatment in eliminating methicillin resistant *Staphylococcus aureus* (MRSA) from diabetic foot infections." *PLoS One* 8: e56022. doi: 10.1371/journal.pone.0056022.

[136] Sanjay, Chhibber; Ashu, Shukla and Sandeep, Kaur. 2017. "Transfersomal Phage Cocktail Is an Effective Treatment against Methicillin-Resistant *Staphylococcus aureus* -Mediated Skin and Soft Tissue Infections." *Antimicrobial Agents chemotherapy* 61: e02146-16. doi: 10.1128/AAC.02146-16.

[137] Wang, Guan H., Bao, Sun F., Xiong, Tuan L., Wang, Yan K., Murfin, Kristen E.,. Xiao, Jin H., Huang, Da W. 2016." Bacteriophage WO Can Mediate Horizontal Gene Transfer in Endosymbiotic *Wolbachia* Genomes." *Frontiers in Microbiology* 7 (1867): 1-16. doi: 10.3389/fmicb.2016.01867.

[138] Kaur, Sandeep., Harjai, Kusum., Chhibber, Sanjay. 2016. "In Vivo Assessment of Phage and Linezolid Based Implant Coatings for Treatment of Methicillin Resistant *S. aureus* (MRSA) Mediated Orthopaedic Device Related Infections." *PLoS One* 11(6): e0157626. doi:10.1371/journal.pone.0157626.

[139] Pincus, Nathan B., Reckhow, Jensen D.; Saleem, Danial; Jammeh, Momodou L.; Datta, Sandip K. and Myles, Ian A. 2015. "Strain Specific Phage Treatment for *Staphylococcus aureus* Infection Is Influenced by Host Immunity and Site of Infection." *PLoS One* 10(4):1-16 e0124280. doi: 10.1371/journal.pone.0124280.

[140] Takemura-Uchiyama, Iyo; Jumpei, Uchiyama; Makoto, Osanai; Norihito, Morimoto; Tadashi, Asagiri; Takako, Ujihara; Masanori, Daibata; Tetsuro, Sugiuraand Shigenobu, Matsuzakiac. 2014. "Experimental phage therapy against lethal lung-derived septicemia caused by *Staphylococcus aureus* in mice." *Microbes and Infection* 6:512-7.

[141] Sue-Er, Hsieh; Hsueh-Hsia, Lo; Shui-Tu, Chen; Mong-Chuan, Lee and Yi-Hsiung, Tseng. 2011. "Wide host range and strong lytic activity of *Staphylococcus aureus* lytic phage Stau2." *Applied of Environmental Microbiology* 77:756–761.

[142] Shigenobu, Matsuzaki; Masaharu, Yasuda; Hiroshi, Nishikawa; Masayuki, Kuroda; Takako, Ujihara; Taro, Shuin; Yuan, Shen; Zhe, Jin; Shigeyoshi, Fujimoto, Nasimuzzaman; Hiroshi, Wakiguchi; Shigeyoshi, Sugihara; Tetsuro, Sugiura; Shigeki, Koda; Asako, Muraoka and Shosuke, Imai. 2003. "Experimental protection of mice against lethal *Staphylococcus aureus* infection by novel bacteriophage φMR11." *The Journal of Infection Disease* 187:613–624.

[143] Mian, Ooi L.; Amanda, Drilling J.; Sandra, Morales; Sandra, Morales; Stephanie, Fong; Sophia, Moraitis; Luis, Macias-Valle; Sarah, Vreugde; Alkis, Psaltis J. and Peter-John, Wormald. 2019. "Safety and Tolerability of Bacteriophage Therapy for Chronic Rhinosinusitis Due to *Staphylococcus aureus.*" *JAMA Otolaryngology Head Neck Surgery* 145:723-729.

[144] Ferry, Tristan., Leboucher, Gilles., Fevre,Cindy., Herry, Yannick., Conrad, Anne., Josse, Jérôme., Batailler, Cécile., Chidiac, Christian., Medina, Lustig, Mathieu S., Laurent, Frédéric., Lyon BJI. 2018. "Salvage debridement, antibiotics and implant retention ("DAIR") with local injection of a selected cocktail of bacteriophages: Is it an option for an elderly patient with relapsing *Staphylococcus aureus* prosthetic-joint infection? *Open Forum Infection Diseases* 5(11): ofy269. doi: 10.1093/ofid/ofy269.

[145] Fish,Randolph., Kutter, Elizabeth., Bryan, Daniel., Wheat, Gordon., Kuhl, Sarah. 2018. "Resolving Digital Staphylococcal Osteomyelitis Using Bacteriophage—A Case Report" *Antibiotics* 7 (87) doi:10.3390/antibiotics7040087.

[146] Fish, R., Kutter, E., Wheat, G., Blasdel, B., Kutateladze, M., Kuhl, S. 2016."Bacteriophage treatment of intransigent diabetic toe ulcers: a case series." *Journal of Wound Care North American Supplement* 25(7): s27-s33.

[147] Fadlallah, Ali; Chelala, Elias and Legeais, Jean-Marc. 2015. "Corneal Infection Therapy with Topical Bacteriophage Administration." *Open Ophthalmology Journal* 4:167-8.

[148] Rhoads, D. D.; Wolcott, R. D.; Kuskowski, M. A.; Wolcott, B. M.; Ward, L. S. and Sulakvelidze, A. 2009. "Bacteriophage therapy of venous leg ulcers in humans: results of a phase I safety trial." *Journal Wound Care* 18:237–238, 240–243.

[149] Gelatti, Luciane C.; Sukiennik, Tereza; Becker, Ana Paula; Inoue, Fernanda M.; do Carmo, Mirian S.; Castrucci, Fernanda M. S.; Pignatari, Antônio C. C.; Ribeiro, Luis C.; Bonamigo, Renan R. and d' Azevedo, Pedro A. 2009. "Sepse por *Staphylococus aureus* resistente à meticilina adquirida na comunidade no sul do Brasil."

Revista da Sociedade Brasileira de Medicina Tropical 42:458-460. [Sepsis by Staphylococcus aureus resistant to methicillin acquired in the community in southern Brazil. *Journal of the Brazilian Society of Tropical Medicine*]

[150] Batista, Cinthia M.; Carvalho, Cícero M. B. and Magalhaes, Nereide S. S. 2007. "Lipossomas e suas aplicações terapêuticas: Estado da arte." *Rev. Bras. Cienc. Farm.* 43(2): 167-179. [Liposomes and their therapeutic applications: State of the art]

[151] Rico, João A. M. 2018 *Nanotecnologia na terapêutica do cancro do pulmão de não pequenas células: a aplicação de lipossoma*. Master diss. Universityof Algarve. http://hdl.handle.net/10400.1/12365. [*Nanotechnology in the treatment of non-small cell lung cancer: the application of liposome*]

[152] Santos, Hercília M. L R. 2005. *Lipossoma convencionais e sítio específico (lectina-conjugada) contendo anaplásicos*. PhD diss. Federal University of Pernambuco. https://repositorio.ufpe.br/bitstream/123456789/2011/1/arquivo5166_1.pdf. [*Conventional liposomes and specific site (lectin-conjugated) containing anaplastics*]

[153] Richa, Singh; Shradhada, Nadhe; Sweeety, Wadhwani; Utkarsha, Shedbalkar and Ananda, Chopad B. 2016. "Nanoparticles for Control of Biofilms *Acinetobacter* Species." *Materials*. 9(5):383. https://www.mdpi.com/1996-1944/9/5/383.

[154] Yuan, Yu-Guo; Peng, Qiu-Ling and Gurunathan, Sangilivandi. 2017. "Effects of silver nanoparticles on multiple drug-resistant strains of *Staphylococcus aureus* and *Pseudomonas aeruginosa* from mastitis-infected goats: an alternative approach forantimicrobial therapy." *Int. J. Mol. Sci.* 18:569. https://www.ncbi.nlm.nih.gov/pubmed/28272303.

[155] Mocan, L.; Matea, Cristian; Tabaran, Flaviu A.; Mosteanu, Ofelia; Pop, Teodora; Puia, Cosmin; Agoston-Coldea, Lucia A; Gonciar, Diana; Kalman, Erszebet; Zaharie, Gabriela; Iancu, CornelandMocan, Teodora. "Selective in vitro photothermal nano-therapy of MRSA

infections mediated by IgG conjugated gold nanoparticles." *Sci Rep.* 6:39466. doi:10.1038/srep39466.

[156] Niemirowicz, Katarzyna; Piktel, Ewelina; Wilczewska, Agnieszka Z.; Markiewicz, Karolina H.; Durnaś, Bonita; Wątek, Marzena; Puszkarz, Irena; Wróblewska, Marta; Niklińska, Wiesława; Savage, Paul B. and Bucki, Robert. 2016 "Core–shell magnetic nanoparticles display synergistic antibacterial effects against *Pseudomonas aeruginosa* and *Staphylococcus aureus* when combined with cathelicidin LL-37 or selected ceragenins." *Int J. Nanomedicine.* 11:5443-5455.

[157] Courtney, Colleen M.; Goodman, Samuel M.; McDaniel, Jessica A.; Madinger, Nancy E.; Chatterjer, Anushree and Nagpal, Prashant. 2016 "Photoexcited quantum dots for killing multidrug-resistant bacteria." *Nature Mater* 15: 529–534.

[158] Allahverdiyev, Adil M.; Kon, Kateryna V.; Abamor, Emrah S.; Bagirova, Malahat and Rafailovich, Miriam 2011. "Coping with antibiotic resistance: combining nanoparticles with antibiotics and other antimicrobial agents." *Expert Rev. Anti. Infect. Ther.* 9:1035–1052.

[159] Chetoni, Patrizia; Burgalassi, Susi; Monti, Daniela; Tampucci, Silvia; Tullio, Vivian; Cuffini, Anna M.; Muntoni, Elisabetta; Spagnolo, Rita; Zara, Gian P. and Cavalli, Roberta. 2016. "Solid lipid nanoparticles as promising tool for intraocular tobramycin delivery: pharmacokinetic studies on rabbits." *Eur. J. Pharm. Biopharm.* 109: 214–223.

[160] Pei, Yihua; Mohamed, Mohamed F.; Seleem, Mohamed N. and Yeo, Yoon. 2017. "Particle engineering for intracellular delivery of vancomycin to methicillin-resistant *Staphylococcus aureus* (MRSA)-infected macrophages." *J. Control. Release* 10: 133–143.

[161] Dizaji, Araz Pen.; Ding, Dan.; Kutsal,; Turk,; Kong, Deling and Piskins, Erhan. 2019. "In vivo imaging/detection of MRSA bacterial infections in mice using fluorescence labelled polymeric nanoparticles carrying vancomycin as the targeting agent." 243: 293-309 https://doi.org/10.1080/09205063.2019.1692631.

[162] Tonga, Chunyi; Zhongb, Xianghua; Yangb, Yuejun; Li, Xu; Zhonga, Guowei; Xiao, Chang. Liu, Bin; Wang, Wei; Yang, Xiaoping. "PB@ PDA@ Ag nanosystem for synergistically eradicating MRSA and accelerating diabetic wound healing assisted with laser irradiation." *Biomaterial.* 243: 11936. https://doi.org/10.1016/j.

[163] Li, Jianghua; Zhong, Wenbin; Zhang, Kaixi; Wang, Dongwei; Hu, Jingbo and Park, Mary B. "Biguanide-Derived Polymeric Nanoparticles Kill MRSA Biofilm and Suppress Infection *In Vivo*." *American Chemical Society*https://dx.doi.org/10.1021/acsami.9b17747.

[164] Kwiatkowakia, Stanislaw; Knapb, Bartosz; Przystupskia, Dawid; Saczkoc, Jolanta; Kedzierkab, Ewa; Knap-Czope, Karoline; Kotinskab, Jolanta; Michelc, Olga; Kottowskia, Krzysztof and Kulback, Julita. 2018. "Photodynamic therapy – mechanisms, fhotosensitizers and combinations." *Biomedicine & Pharmacotherapy.* 106:1098-1107.

[165] Kharkwal, Gitika B.; Sharma, Sulbha K.; Huang, Ying-Ying; Dai, Tianhong and Hamblin, Michael R. 2011 "Photodynamictherapy for infections: clinical applications." *Lasers Surg Med.* 43:755–767.

[166] Allison, Ron R and Moghissi, Keyvan. 2013. "Photodynamic therapy (PDT): PDT mechanisms." *Clin. Endosc.* 46: 24. https://doi.org/10.5946/ce.2013.46.1.24.

[167] Athar, Mohammad, Mukhtar, Hasan, and Bickers, David R. 1988. "Differential role of reactive oxygen intermediates in Photofrin-I- and Photofrin-II mediated hotoenhancement of lipid peroxidation in epidermal microsomal membranes." *J. of Investig. Dermatol.* 90 (5): 652–657.

[168] Redmond, Robert W. and Gamlin, Janet N. 1999. "A compilation of singlet oxygen yields from biologically relevant molecules." *Photochemistry and Photobiology* 70 (4): 391–475.

[169] Fu, Xiu-Jun; Fang, Young and Yao, Min. 2013. "Antimicrobial Photodynamic Therapy for Methicillin-Resistant *Staphylococcus aureus* Infection." *Bio Med Research International* 1-9.

[170] Tubby, Sarah; Wilson, Michael and Nair, Sean P. 2009. "Inactivation of staphylococcal virulence factors using a light-activated antimicrobial agent." *BMC Microbiology*. 9 (211) https://doi.org/10.1186/1471-2180-9-211.

[171] Freitas, Mirian AA; Pereira, André H. C.; Pinto, Juliana G.; Casas, Adriana and Ferreira-Strixino, Juliana. 2019. "Bacterial viability after antimicrobial photodynamic therapy with curcumin on multiresistant *Staphylococcus aureus*." *Future Microbiol*. 14(9): 739–748.

[172] Scheinfeld, Noan. 2015. "The use of photodynamic therapy to treat hidradenitis suppurativa a review and critical analysis." *Dermatology Online Journal* 21: 1-5.

[173] Dweba, Cwengile C.,Zishiri, Oliver T. and Zowalaty, Mohamed E. E. 2018. "Methicillin-resistant *Staphylococcus aureus*: livestock-associated, antimicrobial, and heavy metal resistance." *Infect Drug Resist*. 11: 2497–2509.

[174] Braz, Márcia; Salvador, Diana; Gomes, Ana T. P. C.; Mesquita, Mariana Q.; Faustino, Maria A. F.; Neves, Maria G. P. M. S. and Almeida, Adelaide. 2020. "Photodynamic inactivation of methicillin-resistant *Staphylococcus aureus* on skin using a porphyrinic formulation." *Photodiagnosis Photodyn Ther*. 23:101754. doi: 10.1016/j.pdpdt.2020.101754.

[175] Schreiner, M.; Bäumler, W.; Eckl, D. B.; Späth, A.; König, B. and Eichner, A. 2018. "Photodynamic inactivation of bacteria to decolonize meticillin-resistant *Staphylococcus aureus* from human skin." *British Journal of Dermatology* 179: 1358–1367.

[176] Tasl, Hüseyin; Akbıyık, Ayşe; Topaloğlu, Nermin; Alptuzun, Vildan and Parlar, Sulunay. 2018. "Photodynamic antimicrobial activity of new porphyrin derivatives against methicillin resistant *Staphylococcus aureus.*" *Journal of Microbiology* 56(11): 828–837.

[177] Makdoumi, Karim; Hedin, Marie and Bäckman, Anders. 2018. "Different photodynamic effects of blue light with and without riboflavin on methicillin-resistant *Staphylococcus aureus* (MRSA) and human keratinocytes *in vitro*." *Lasers in Medical Science*. https://doi.org/10.1007/s10103-019-02774-9.

[178] Iqbal, Gulrukh; Faisal, Sulaiman; Khan, Sara; Shams, Dilawar F.; Nadhman, Akhtar. 2019. "Photo-inactivation and efflux pump inhibition of methicillin resistant *Staphylococcus aureus* using thiolated cobalt doped ZnO nanoparticles." *Journal of Photochemistry & Photobiology, B: Biology* 192: 141–146.

[179] Wong, Tak-Wah Liao, Shu-Zhen; Ko, Wen-Chien; Wu, Chi-Jung; Wu, Shin B.; Chuang, Yin-Ching and Huang, I-Hsiu. 2019. "Indocyanine Green mediated photodynamic therapy reduces methicillin-resistant *Staphylococcus aureus*. Drug Resistance." *J Clin Med.* 8(3):411-20.

[180] Santos, Denisar P.; Lopes, Diego P. S.; Calado, Stefano P. M.; Gonçalves, Caroline V.; Muniz, Igor P. R.; Ribeiro, Israel S.;Galantini, Maria P. L. and Silva, Robson A. A. 2019. "Efficacy of photoactivated *Myrciaria cauliflora* extract against *Staphylococcus aureus* infection - A pilot study." *J. Photochem. Photobiol. B.* 191:107-115.

[181] Walter, Alec B.; Simpson, Jocelyn; Jenkins, Logan J.;Skaar, Eric P. and Jansen, Duco E. 2020. "Optimization of optical parameters for improved photodynamic therapy of *Staphylococcus aureus* using endogenous coproporphyrin III." *Photodiagnosis Photodyn Ther* 29:101624.

[182] Texeira, Marcus Z. 2007. "Homeopatia: prática médica humanística." *Rev. Assoc. Med. Bras.* 53: 6 - 10.

[183] Rattanachaikunsopon, Pongsak and Phumkhachorm, Parichat. 2010. "Antimicrobial activity of Basil (*Ocimum basilicum*) oil against *Salmonella enteritidis in vitro* and food." *Biosci. Biotecnol. Biochem.* 23: 74-6.

[184] Fisher, Peter. et al. 2005. "Are the clinical effects of homoeopathy placebo effects?" *Lancet* 366: 2082–2083.

[185] Linde, Klaus; Clausius, Nicola and Ramirez, Gilbert. 1997. "Are the clinical effects of homeopathy placebo effects? A meta-analysis of placebo-controlled trials." *Lancet* 350: 834–843.

[186] Smith, Cyril W. 2015. "Electromagnetic and magnetic vector potential bio-information and water." *Homeopathy* 104(04): 301-304.

[187] Milgrom, Lionel R. 2005. "The sound of two hands clapping: Could homeopathy work locally and non-locally?" *Homeopathy* 94: 100–104.

[188] Almirantis, Yannis. 2013. "Homeopathy e between tradition and modern science: remedies as carriers of significance." *Homeopathy* 102: 114-122.

[189] Clausen, Jürgen; van Wijk, Roeland and Albrecht, Henning. 2010. "Infection models in basic research on homeopathy." *Homeopathy* 99: 263-270.

[190] Nascimento, Katia F. et al. 2017. "M1 homeopathic complex trigger effective responses against *Leishmania amazonensis in vivo* and *in vitro*." *Cytokine* 99: 80–90.

[191] Cajueiro, Ana P. B. et al. 2017. "Homeopathic medicines cause Th1 predominance and induce spleen and megakaryocytes changes in BALB/c mice infected with *Leishmania infantum*." *Cytokine* 95:97-101.

[192] Passeti, Tânia A. et al. 2014. "Ação dos medicamentos homeopáticos *Arnica montana, Gelsemium sempervirens, Belladonna, Mercurius solubillis* e nosódio sobre o crescimento *"in vitro"* da bactéria *Streptococcus pyogenes*." *Rev. Homeop.* 77(1/2): 1- 9. [Action of homeopathic medicines *Arnica montana, Gelsemium sempervirens, Belladonna, Mercurius solubillis* and nosode on the "in vitro" growth of the bacterium *Streptococcus pyogenes*.]

[193] Pannek, Jürgen. et al. 2018. *In vitro* Effects of Homeopathic Drugs on Cultured *Escherichia coli*. *Homeopathy* 107(2):150-154.

[194] Clinical Laboratory Standard Institute (CLSI). *Performance standards for antimicrobial susceptibility testing*. Seventeenth Information Supplement M 100-S24. Wayne, Pennsylvania: CLSI, 2014.

[195] Gerstel, Johanne; Turner, Tiffany; Ruiz, Guillermo; Wise, Justin; Stein, Ashley; Jones, Greg; Morin, Tanya; Pinazza, Tony; Sukhorukov, Elena; Clark, Donna; Steen, Taelor; Wright, Berlin and Langland, Jeffrey. 2018. "Identification of botanicals with potential

therapeutic use against methicillin-resistant *Staphylococcus aureus* (MRSA) infections." *Phytotherapy Research* 1–9.

[196] Paglia, Adriano P. and Pinto, Luiz P. 2010. "Biodiversidade da mata atlântica. In: E. Marone, D. Riet, & T. Melo. Brasil Atlântico - um país com a raiz na mata." *Instituto Bio Atlântica* 102-129.

[197] Gatadi, Srikanth; Gour, Jitendra and Nanduri, Srinivas. 2019 "Natural product derived promising anti-MRSA drug leads: A review." *Bioorganic & Medicinal Chemistry* 27: 3760–3774.

[198] Barbosa, Deysi C. S. and Correia, Maria T. S.2015. "Potencial antibiótico de extratos alcoólicos de plantas da região da caatinga contra bactérias multirresistentes." *XXIII CONIC – Congresso de Iniciação Científica.* Accessed March, 12, 2019. https://www.ufpe.br/documents/616030/858617/Potencial_antibiotico_de_extratos_alcoolicos.pdf. [Antibiotic potential of alcoholic extracts of plants from the caatinga region against multi-resistant bacteria. *XXIII CONIC - Scientific Initiation Congress.*]

[199] Siqueira, Anderson L.; Dantas, Camila G.; Gomes, Margarete Z.; Padilha, Francine F.; Albuquerque Jr., Ricardo L. C. and Cardoso, Juliana C. 2014. "Estudo da ação antibacteriana do extrato hidroalcoólico de própolis vermelha sobre *Enterococcus faecalis.*" *Rev Odontol UNESP* 43(6): 359-366. [Study of the antibacterial action of the hydroalcoholic extract of red propolis on *Enterococcus faecalis. Rev Odontol UNESP*]

[200] Kuok, Chiu-Fai; Hoi, Sai-On; Hoi, Chi-Fai; Chan, Chi-Hong; Fong, Io-Hong; Ngok, Cheong-Kei; Meng, Li-Rong and Fong, Pedro. 2017. "Synergistic antibacterial effects of herbal extracts and antibiotics on methicillin-resistant *Staphylococcus aureus*: A computational and experimental study." *Experimental Biology and Medicine* 242: 731–743.

[201] Cruz-Sáncheza, Natividad G.; Gómez-Riverab, Abraham, Alvarez-Fitzc, Patricia; Ventura-Zapatad, Elsa; Pérez-García, Ma Dolores; Avilés-Florese, Margarida; Gutiérrez-Romána, Ana S. and González-Cortazar, Manasés. 2019. "Antibacterial activity of *Morinda citrifolia* Linneo seeds against *Methicillin-Resistant Staphylococcus spp.*" *Microbial Pathogenesis* 128: 347–353.

[202] Hossion, Abugafar M. L.; Zamami, Yoshito; Kandahary, Rafiya K.; Tsuchiya, Tomofusa; Ogawa, Wakano; Iwado, Akimasa; Sasaki, Kenji. 2011. "Quercetin diacylglycoside analogues showing dual inhibition of DNA gyrase and topoisomerase IV as novel antibacterial agents." *J Med Chem.*, 54:3686–3703.

[203] Vivas, Roberto; Barbosa, Ana A. T.; Dolabela, Silvia S.; and Jain, Sona. 2019. "Multidrug-Resistant Bacteria and Alternative methods to Control Them: An Overview." *Microbial Drug Resistance* 0:1-19.

[204] Rai, Mahendra; Paralikar, Priti; Jogee, Priti; Agarkar, Gauravi; Ingle, Avinash P.; Derita, Marcos and Zacchino, Susana. 2017. "Synergistic antimicrobial potential of essential oils in combination with nanoparticles: emerging trends and future perspectives." *Int. J. Pharm.* 519:67–78.

[205] Ghaderi, L., Moghimi, R., Aliahmadi, A., McClements, D. J., and Rafati, H. 2017. "Development of antimicrobial nanoemulsion-based delivery systems against selected pathogenic bacteria using a thymol rich *Thymus daenensis* essential oil." *J. Appl. Microbiol.* 123:832–840.

[206] Altieri, Karen T.; Sanitá, Paula V.; Machado, Ana L.; Giampaolo, Eunice T.; Pavarina, Ana C.; Jorge, Janaina H. and Vergani, Carlos E. 2013. "Eradication of a Mature Methicillin-Resistant *Staphylococcus aureus* (MRSA) Biofilm from Acrylic Surfaces." *Braz. Dent. J.* 24: 5-12.

[207] Selvaraj, Antonymuthu; Jayasree, Tangaraj; Valliammai, Alaguvel and Pandian, Shunmugiah K. (2019). "Mytenol attenuates MRSA Biofilm and virulence by suppressing *sarA* expression." *Dynamism. from Microbiol.* 4:10-20.

BIOGRAPHICAL SKETCHES

Susana Nogueira Diniz

Affiliation: Anhanguera University of Sao Paulo, São Paulo, Brazil

Education: Doctorate degree in Biochemistry and Immunology

Research and Professional Experience: Molecular and cellular immunology, Microbiology, biomarker, immunoregulation.

Professional Appointments: Graduated in Biology from the Federal University of Minas Gerais (1993) with a master's degree and PhD in Molecular Biology, in the area of applied Immunology and Microbiology, at the Federal University of Minas Gerais (2001). Has been in the academics field since 2008 being the leader of the Laboratory of Molecular Biology and Functional Genomics at Anhanguera University of São Paulo in Brazil. Has worked with research based on the interaction between the areas of products and technological bioprocesses in health. In this way, the works carried out by her group are aimed at generating technologies based on aspects of cellular and molecular for use and application in animal and human health.

Publications from the Last 3 Years:

Civa, Maéli M. F.; Souza, Dirceu G. De; Silva, Renata G.; Maciel, Dayany Da S. A.; Tranquilin, Ricardo L.; Diniz, Susana N.; Okuyama, Cristina E.; Santos, Márcio L. Dos; Pereira, Regina M. S. . Metal Complexes Derived of Diosmin with Biological Activities *in vitro*. *Journal of Materials Science Research*, v. 9, p. 10, 2019.

Diniz, Susana N.; Marquez, A. S.; Costa, N. M. L.; Okuyama, C. E. . Perspectivas de Abordagem da Bioética na Educação Básica. *Revista De Ensino, Educação E Ciências Humanas*, v. 19, p. 227, 2018. doi.org/10.17921/2447-8733.2018v19n2p227-232. [Perspectives of

Bioethics Approach in Basic Education. *Journal of Teaching, Education and Human Sciences*]

Gema, S.; Oliveira, E. M. L.; Okuyama, C. E.; Diniz, S. N. Parâmetros clínicos, biológicos e moleculares na resposta ao tratamento com interferon-beta em pacientes com esclerose múltipla. *Enciclopédia Biosfera*, v. 15, p. 1261-1279, 2018. DOI: 10.18677/EnciBio_2018B100. [Clinical, biological and molecular parameters in response to treatment with interferon-beta in patients with multiple sclerosis. *Biosphere Encyclopedia*]

Monteiro, Jordana; Monteiro, Rodrigo; Okuyama, Cristina; Diniz, Susana . A importância da analgesia e do uso de anti-inflamatórios não esteroidais cox2 seletivos na prevenção e tratamento do câncer em cães. *Enciclopédia Biosfera*, v. 16, p. 29-48, 2019. 10.18677/EnciBio_2019A3. [The importance of analgesia and the use of selective cox2 nonsteroidal anti-inflammatory drugs in the prevention and treatment of cancer in dogs. *Biosphere Encyclopedia*]

Pinheiro, Marcelo Maia, Pinheiro, Felipe Moura Maia, Resende, Ludmilla Lp Amaral, Diniz, Susana Nogueira, Andrea Fabbri, Marco Infante, Improvement of pure sensory mononeuritis multiplex and IgG1deficiency with sitagliptin and vitamin D3. European *Review for medical and pharmacological science*. 2020 (accepted).

Radunz Cl, Okuyama Ce, Branco-Barreiro Fca, Pereira Rms, Diniz Sn. Clinical randomized trial study of hearing aids effectiveness in association with Ginkgo biloba extract (EGb761) on tinnitus improvement. *Braz J Otorhinolaryngol*. 786: 1 1-9. 2019.

Tânia Aguiar Passeti

Affiliation: Anhanguera University of Sao Paulo, São Paulo, Brazil

Education: PhD in Immunology

Research and Professional Experience: Immunology, experimental pathology, biological activity of plant extracts and homeopathy in microbiology.

Professional Appointments: - Graduation in Pharmacy-Biochemistry Oswaldo Cruz college (1988), Master in Clinical Analysis from the Faculty of Pharmaceutical Sciences of the University of São Paulo (1993) and PhD in Immunology Sciences, from the Institute of Biomedical Sciences of the University of São Paulo - ICBUSP (1997). Part of the PhD in Institut fur Experimentelle Dermatologie, Germany (1994). Post-doctorate at the Anhanguera University of São Paulo - UNIAN in action of homeopathic medicines on microorganisms and biological activity of plant extracts. Extensive experience in university teaching in the courses of Medicine, Pharmacy, Physiotherapy, Biomedicine, Veterinary Medicine, Nursing and Occupational Therapy. Competence in the disciplines of Pathology, Microbiology, Immunology and Physiology.

Honors: - Award in the category "Reducción", III Congresso Latino Americano de Métodos Alternativos (2018). Honorable Mention in XI Congresso Brasileiro de Farmácia Homeopática. Associação Brasileira de Farmacêuticos Homeopáticas (2017).

Publications from the Last 3 Years:

Araujo, M. E.; Araujo, C. G. C.; Armando Junior, J.; Passeti, A. T. Ação do extrato aquoso de Quercus sp. sobre o crescimento in vitro da bactéria *Escherichia coli*. *Interação* (São Paulo- Brazil – ISSN: 2357-7975), v. 1, p. 140-143, 2018. [Action of the aqueous extract of Quercus sp. on the in vitro growth of the bacteria *Escherichia coli. Interaction*]

Passeti, A. T.; Coelho, C. P.; Bonamin, L. V. Chapter 8 - High dilution: changing the future infection? *Transdisciplinanarity and Translationality in High Dilution Research*. 1ed. British: Cambridge Scholars, 2019, v. 1, p. 130-139.

Audrey de Souza Marquez

Affiliation: Center of Research in Health Sciences. University of Northern Paraná, UNOPAR Londrina, PR, BR

Education: Doctorate degree in Microbiology

Research and Professional Experience: Microbiology, immunology, paracoccidioidomycosis, inflammatory markers, vitamin D and ageing.

Professional Appointments: Graduated in pharmacy-Biochemistry from the State University of Londrina (1994) with a master's degree and PhD in Microbiology, in the area of applied Immunology, at the State University of Londrina (2007) and MBA in Project Management by Fundação Getúlio Vargas (2014). Has been in the medical diagnosis field since 1995 and in academics since 2000. Has worked as Director of Technical Issues and Research at CETEL Laboratory, Director of Center of Research in Health Sciences and Coordinator of the Committee on Ethics in Research at Unopar University. Currently, performs as Supervisor of Quality and Scientific Advice of Sabin-Diagnostic Medicine Laboratory and as Coordinator of the Collegiate of Ethics in Research of Kroton Educacional. Develops research in the topics: paracoccidioidomycosis, inflammatory markers, vitamin D and aging.

Honors: "Nossa Gente de Londrina" (JL Jornal de Londrina prize) award nominated for the EELO project (Study on Ageing and Longevity), in 2014.

Publications from the Last 3 Years:

Déborah C. D. S. Caetano; Cristina E. Okuyama; Márcia R. M. Dos Santos; Audrey De S. Marquez; Susana N. Diniz; Regina M. S. Pereira. Tegumentary leishmaniasis in Brazil: socio-demographic and health characteristics associated with laboratory and electrocardiographic adverse reactions. *Ensaios e Ciência*, 2020 (Submitted).

Oliveira, Denise Cristine De; Okuyama, Cristina Eunice; Fernandes, Karen Barros Parron; Poli-Frederico, Regina Célia; Diniz, Susana Nogueira; Costa, Viviane De Souza Pinho; Marquez, Audrey De Souza. The importance of recommended 25-hydroxyvitamin D levels in the glycemic control of diabetic elderly: From the Study on Aging and Longevity (EELO) project. *Maturitas*, 2020. (Submitted)

Bazoni, Jessica Aparecida; Ciquinato, Daiane Soares Almeida; Marquez, Audrey De Souza; Costa, Viviane De Souza Pinho; Marchiori, Glória De Moraes; Marchiori, Luciana Lozza De Moraes. Hypovitaminosis D, Low Bone Mineral Density, and Diabetes Mellitus as Probable Risk Factors for Benign Paroxysmal Positional Vertigo in the Elderly. *International Archives of Otorhinolaryngology* (PRINT), v. 2, p. 9-12, 2019.

Cezar-Dos-Santos, Fernando; Lenhard-Vidal, Adriane; Assolini, João Paulo; Marquez, A. S.; Ono, Mário Augusto; Itano, Eiko Nakagawa. *Paracoccidioides restrepiensis* B339 (PS3) and P. lutzii LDR2 yeast cells and soluble components display in vitro hemolytic and hemagglutinating activities on human erythrocytes. *Microbiology and Immunology*, v. 62, p. 436-443, 2018.

Everton Tadeu Prado

Affiliation: Anhanguera University of Sao Paulo, Sao Paulo, Brazil

Education: Master's degree in pharmacy

Research and Professional Experience: Microbiology, Clinical Analysis Laboratory and University Teacher.

Publications from the Last 3 Years:

Karen Cristiane Higa, Adeline Lacerda Jorjão, Simone Aparecida Biazzi De Lapena, Everton Tadeu Prado, Fernanda Malagutti Tomé, Andreia Ferreira Diniz Cortelli, Viviane Borio Conceição, Priscila Ebram De Miranda, Luciane Dias De Oliveira. Cytotoxic and antiinflamatory activity of the glycolic extract of camellia sinensis (l.) kuntze in lps-stimulated machrophages (RAW 264.7). *Braz. J. Hea. Rev.*, Curitiba, v. 3, n. 1, p. 1094-1108 jan./feb. 2020. DOI: https://doi.org/10.34119/bjhrv3n1-085.

Claudia Forlin da Silva

Affiliation: Anhanguera University of Sao Paulo, São Paulo, Brazil

Education: PhD student in Biotechnology and Health Innovation

Research and Professional Experience: Intensivist Nurse and Neonatologist, University Teacher

Publications from the Last 3 Years:

Forlin. C.; Diniz, S. N. The technological / market prospecting of ATS. In: Meeting of Scientific Activities, 2019, Londrina-Pr. *Proceedings of the Scientific Activities Meeting*. Londrina-PR: Unopar, 2019. v. E56a.

Forlin. C.; Galleguillos, T. G. B. The pedagogical structure of the nursing course at a higher education institution in the city of São Paulo - Brazil. In: *XIII National Research Seminar and XVI Scientific Initiation Meeting of Uninove, 2019, São Paulo. Scientific Initiation Meeting*. São Paulo: Nove de Julho University (Uninove), 2019. v. XIII. P. 48-52.

Danielli dos Santos Baeta

Affiliation: São Paulo State University (Unesp), School of Pharmaceutical Sciences, Araraquara

Education: PhD in Biotechnology

Research and Professional Experience: Biochemistry, enzymes and biochemical studies of fruits

Katia Sivieri

Affiliation: Anhanguera University of Sao Paulo, São Paulo, Brazil

Education: PhD in Food technology

Research and Professional Experience: Microbiology, food microbiology and gut microbiota

Publications from the Last 3 Years:

Bianchi, F; Lopes, N. P.; Adorno, M. A. T.; Sakamoto, I. K.; Genovese, M. I.; Saad, S. M. I.; Sivieri, K. Impact of combining acerola by-product with a probiotic strain on a gut microbiome model. *International Journal of Food Sciences and Nutrition*, v. 69, p. 1-10, 2018.

Bianchi, Fernanda; Duque, Ana Luiza Rocha Faria; Saad, Susana Marta Isay; Sivieri, Katia. Gut microbiome approaches to treat obesity in humans. *Applied Microbiology and Biotechnology*, v. 103, p. 1081-1094, 2019.

Bianchi, Fernanda; Larsen, Nadja; De Mello Tieghi, Thatiana; Adorno, Maria Angela Tallarico; Kot, Witold; Saad, Susana Marta Isay; Jespersen, Lene; Sivieri, Katia. Modulation of gut microbiota from obese individuals by *in vitro* fermentation of citrus pectin in combination with Bifidobacterium longum BB-46. *Applied Microbiology and Biotechnology*, v. 102, p. 8827-8840, 2018.

Bianchi, Fernanda; Larsen, Nadja; Tieghi, Thatiana De Mello; Adorno, Maria Angela T.; Saad, Susana M.I.; Jespersen, Lene; Sivieri, Katia. *In vitro* modulation of human gut microbiota composition and metabolites by Bifidobacterium longum BB-46 and a citric pectin. *Food Research International*, v. 120, p. 595-602, 2018.

Brito, Sabrina Da Costa; Bresolin, Joana D; Sivieri, Kátia; Ferreira, Marcos D. Low-density polyethylene films incorporated with silver nanoparticles to promote antimicrobial efficiency in food packaging. *Food Science and Technology International*, v. 27, p. 108201321989420-10, 2019.

Cárdenas-Castro, Alicia Paulina; Bianchi, Fernanda; Tallarico-Adorno, María Angela; Montalvo-González, Efigenia; Sáyago-Ayerdi, Sonia G.; Sivieri, Katia. *In vitro* colonic fermentation of Mexican -taco- from corn-tortilla and black beans in a Simulator of Human Microbial Ecosystem (SHIME®) system. *Food Research International*, v. 118, p. 81-88, 2018.

Fidélix, Melaine Priscila; Milenkovic, Dragan; Cesar, Thais; Sivieri, Katia. Microbiota modulation and effects on metabolic biomarkers by orange juice: a controlled clinical trial. *Food & Function*, v. 11, p. 1599-1610, 2020.

Lima, Ana Carolina Delgado; Cecatti, Clara; Fidélix, Melaine Priscila; Adorno, Maria Angela Tallarico; Sakamoto, Isabel Kimiko; Cesar, Thais Borges; Sivieri, Katia. Effect of Daily Consumption of Orange Juice on the Levels of Blood Glucose, Lipids, and Gut Microbiota Metabolites: Controlled Clinical Trials. *Journal of Medicinal Food*, v. 22, p. 1-12, 2019.

Rodrigues, Vivian Cristina Da Cruz; Duque, Ana Luiza Rocha Faria; Fino, Luciana De Carvalho; Simabuco, Fernando Moreira; Sartoratto, Adilson; Cabral, Lucélia; Noronha, Melline Fontes; Sivieri, Katia; Antunes, Adriane Elisabete Costa. Modulation of the intestinal microbiota and the metabolites produced by the administration of ice cream and a dietary supplement containing the same probiotics. *British Journal of Nutrition*, v. 1, p. 1-36, 2020.

Salgaço, Mateus Kawata; Oliveira, Liliane Garcia Segura; Costa, Giselle Nobre; Bianchi, Fernanda; Sivieri, Katia. Relationship between gut microbiota, probiotics, and type 2 diabetes mellitus. *Applied Microbiology and Biotechnology*, v. 1, p. 1-10, 2019.

Chapter 2

METHICILLIN-RESISTANT *STAPHYLOCOCCUS AUREUS*: OLD AND NEW THERAPEUTIC APPROACHES

Sandrelli Meridiana de Fátima Ramos dos Santos Medeiros[1], MD, Iago Dillion Lima Cavalcanti[1], MD, Ketly Rodrigues Barbosa dos Anjos[2], Mariane Cajubá de Britto Lira Nogueira[1,3], PhD and Isabella Macário Ferro Cavalcanti[1,2,], PhD*

[1]Laboratory of Immunopathology Keizo Asami (LIKA), Federal University of Pernambuco (UFPE), Recife, PE, Brazil
[2]Laboratory of Microbiology and Immunology, Federal University of Pernambuco/Academic Center of Vitória (UFPE/CAV), Vitória de Santo Antão, PE, Brazil
[3]Laboratory of Nanotechnology, Biotechnology and Cell Culture (NanoBioCel), Federal University of Pernambuco/Academic Center of Vitória (UFPE/CAV), Vitória de Santo Antão, PE, Brazil

---

* Corresponding Author's E-mail: isabella.cavalcanti@ufpe.br; bel_macario@yahoo.com.br.

ABSTRACT

Staphylococcus aureus is a microorganism that presents several virulence factors besides the ability to acquire resistance to a large number of antibiotics. The clinical and indiscriminate use of methicillin allowed the appearance of methicillin-resistant *S. aureus* (MRSA), considered one of the leading causes of nosocomy infections, with high mortality rates worldwide. The pattern of antimicrobial susceptibility and the prevalence of this pathogen varies widely between countries and regions. Infections caused by this microorganism result in a hospital stay increase and high costs associated with medical care. Also, infections caused by MRSA that were previously associated only with hospital environments can already be found in the community infecting people without predisposing risk factors. Therefore, MRSA is not only seen as a nosocomial pathogen. Besides, the prevalence and epidemiology of MRSA are continually changing, with new MRSA strains appearing in different geographic regions. Regarding the therapy, vancomycin has been historically the standard drug for treatment, and sometimes the last resort for the treatment of severe MRSA infections, providing empirical coverage and definitive treatment. However, its indiscriminate use led to the development of vancomycin-resistant *S. aureus* (VRSA). In this sense, this book chapter seeks to describe the main available therapeutic possibilities for the treatment of MRSA/VRSA infections and the new therapeutic approaches that demonstrate efficacy in scientific research and arouse interest in the medical area.

Keywords: MRSA, VRSA, vancomycin, new therapy approaches.

INTRODUCTION

Staphylococcus aureus was first identified as bacterial pathogens in the 19th century (Lakhundi; Zhang, 2018). *S. aureus* is considered an opportunistic human pathogen and is often associated with infections acquired in the community and the hospital environment (Taylor; Unakal, 2019). It is responsible for acute infections that can spread to different tissues and can progress to more severe diseases such as pneumonia, osteomyelitis, endocarditis, among others (Reddy; Srirama; Dirisala, 2017).

Currently, one of the major clinical concerns for *S. aureus* infections is its resistance profile known as methicillin-resistant *S. aureus* (MRSA), being responsible for the high mortality rates (Raygada; Levine, 2009, Taylor; Unakal, 2019). The resistance of MRSA strains is related to changes in penicillin-binding proteins, encoded by the *mecA* gene, without being related to the production of beta-lactamase. Due to the presence of these proteins, methicillin and penicillinase-resistant compounds have a low affinity for the bacteria site of action (Baek et al., 2014).

MRSA is one of the main causes of infections acquired in hospitals and is commonly associated with morbidity, mortality, length of stay, and high costs. Besides, MRSA can cause severe and fatal infections such as bloodstream infection, infective endocarditis, pneumonia, skin, and tissue infections. MRSA infections can be categorized into hospital-associated (HA-MRSA) and community-associated (CA-MRSA) MRSA infections. Recently, a new type of MRSA that arose from animals designated livestock-associated MRSA (LA-MRSA) was described (Boswihi; Udo, 2018; Lakhundi; Zhang, 2018; Costa-Junior et al., 2019). The different types differ not only to their clinical features and molecular biology, but also on their antibiotic susceptibility and treatment (Cadena et al., 2016; Palavecino, 2020).

There are several antibiotics applied in the treatment of infections caused by *S. aureus*. It can be cited as example methicillin, vancomycin, rifampicin, clindamycin, linezolid, among others. Currently, with the emergence of resistant strains, induced by inadequate antibiotic choices, or even their misuse, there are few antibiotic options on the market (Luna et al., 2010). Penicillins were recognized as the drugs of choice until *S. aureus* developed penicillin resistance by the production of beta-lactamase (Lakhundi; Zhang, 2018).

Antibiotic resistance has become a major health problem, with the inactivation of the main options for the treatment of *S. aureus* infections. Penicillins- resistant strains were the first strains to emerge, and nowadays, there are resistant strains to practically all classes of antibiotics used to supply the ineffectiveness of penicillins. It is the case of vancomycin, which emerged as an alternative in the treatment of MRSA infections there are already strains of vancomycin-intermediate *S. aureus* (VISA) and vancomycin-resistant *S. aureus* (VRSA) (Luna et al., 2010; Liu et al., 2011).

MRSA infections have created an urgent need to discover new therapeutic alternatives for this resistance profile. Due to the high incidence and mortality rate of MRSA infections, the necessity for alternatives to circumvent this resistance has become a public health problem (Lakhundi; Zhang, 2018; Gatadi; Gour; Nanduri, 2019). Many innovative strategies for the development of alternative drugs are being adopted, including the interruption of biofilms, bacteriophage-derived antimicrobials, anti-staphylococcal vaccines, as well as the development of nanosystems aiming the encapsulation of antimicrobials (Grunenwald; Bennett; Skaar, 2019). In this sense, this book chapter seeks to describe the main available therapeutic options for the treatment of MRSA/VRSA infections and the new therapeutic approaches that demonstrate efficacy in scientific research and arouse interest in the medical area.

STAPHYLOCOCCUS AUREUS

Staphylococcus aureus: Infection and Virulence Profile

Staphylococcus aureus is a spherical-shaped bacterium belonging to the gram-positive group. It tends to organize in clusters that are described as "grape curls," in which their colonies are usually golden or yellow. *Staphylococcus aureus* grows at temperatures between 18 and 40 °C and may grow in an aerobic or anaerobic environment (Santos et al., 2007; Taylor; Unakal, 2019).

The identification tests of *S. aureus* include positive catalase, positive coagulase, susceptibility to novobiocin, and fermentation of the mannitol (Santos et al., 2007; Taylor; Unakal, 2019). Also, tests are conducted to verify acetoin production for differentiation between *Staphylococcus aureus*, *Staphylococcus hyicus*, *Staphylococcus delphini* and *Staphylococcus intermedius* (Ferreira et al., 2006). *S. aureus* is present mainly in the skin and nasal pits of healthy people, as well as may also be present in animals and food (Taylor; Unakal, 2019). It is estimated that 30 to 60% of the healthy human individuals are colonized with *S. aureus* and are conducive to developing some type of infection which can range from skin infections to life-threatening infections such as pneumonias, sepsis, and endocarditis (Bes et al., 2018; Mandel et al., 2018). *S. aureus* is considered the most common microorganism in blood infections, and despite the use of antimicrobials, it has a high mortality rate (Kim et al., 2018). Its transmission can occur through direct contact between people, being widespread transmission in hospital environments (Sales; Silva, 2012; Bes et al., 2018).

In addition to infections, *S. aureus* can cause specific conditions due to the production of toxins such as scalding skin syndrome, staphylococcal food poisoning, and toxic shock syndrome (Schmidt; Kock; Ehelers, 2017).

Scalding skin syndrome occurs due to the production of two exotoxins that bind to the epidermis, causing disruption of protective barriers of the skin and facilitating infections by *S. aureus* (Mishra; Yadav; Mishra, 2016). Exotoxins are also responsible for the development of toxic shock syndrome, which is characterized as a self-inflammatory process induced by the immune system in response to infection, leading to severe dysfunction of multiple organs and systems, presenting a rapid and progressive clinical course (Marton, 2016).

S. aureus is commonly associated with food poisoning due to its frequent presence in food. Food poisoning is due to the ingestion of preformed staphylococcal enterotoxins in food, and its diagnosis is confirmed by counting *S. aureus* higher than 10^5 CFU g^{-1} present in food remains or by the detection of enterotoxins (Werlang et al., 2019).

The success of *S. aureus* as a pathogen is attributable, partly the diversity of virulence factors produced, since they facilitate the invasion and colonization of the host tissue, the evasion of the immune defense mechanisms of the host, aid in the acquisition and the spread of bacteria in the host tissue. Due to the full range of virulence factors produced are numerous enzymes and cytotoxins, such as coagulase, collagenase, exfoliative toxins, hemolysins, hyaluronidase, leukocidin, lipases, nucleases, and staphylocycins, in addition to the capacity to produce biofilm (Schmidt; Kock; Ehlers, 2017).

Biofilm can be defined as multicellular structures formed by the binding and aggregation of microorganisms, followed by the coating with an extracellular matrix rich in polysaccharides (Costa et al., 2018). The production of biofilm by bacteria increases the potential for adherence of these microorganisms on several surfaces. Thus they are considered a factor of virulence because it is a defense system used by bacteria against the immune system of animals and in the action of antimicrobial agents (Araújo et al., 2017).

Treatment of Infections Caused by *Staphylococcus aureus*

Treatment using antimicrobials is an essential step in controlling infections caused by *S. aureus* (Kim et al., 2019). To define the most adequate treatment, it is necessary to understand the characteristics and epidemiology of the pathogen (Troeman; Van Hout; Kluytmans, 2019). Studies show that most infections caused by *S. aureus* are induced by the bacterial microbiota of the patient himself (endogenous infections) or develop after the exogenous acquisition of the environment or other people (Von Eiff et al., 2001; Kao et al., 2015).

One circumstance that turns it very difficult to treat *S. aureus* infections is that there are phenotypic and genotypic variations, showing a genetic heterogeneity in populations of *S. aureus*. These variations can be identified based on biochemical characteristics and antimicrobial sensitivity (Alfouzan et al., 2019).

Vancomycin is the most used medicine for the treatment of infections caused by *S. aureus* (Liu et al., 2011; Damasco et al., 2019). However, other medicines can be applied in the treatment of these infections, such as rifampicin, clindamycin, oxacillin, linezolid, tigecycline, daptomycin, aminoglycosides, fluoroquinolones, macrolides, and trimethoprim-sulfamethoxazole. The choice of the best treatment will depend on the strain susceptibility to the available antibiotics (Bhattacharya et al., 2015; Ansari et al., 2019).

Despite a large number of antibiotics currently present on the market, their inadequate use can result in bacterial resistance, causing recurrence of infection and causing severe complications (Horino; Hori, 2019; Kim et al., 2019). The ability of a bacterium to resist the action of antibiotics is defined as bacterial resistance (Figure 1) (Li; Webster, 2018).

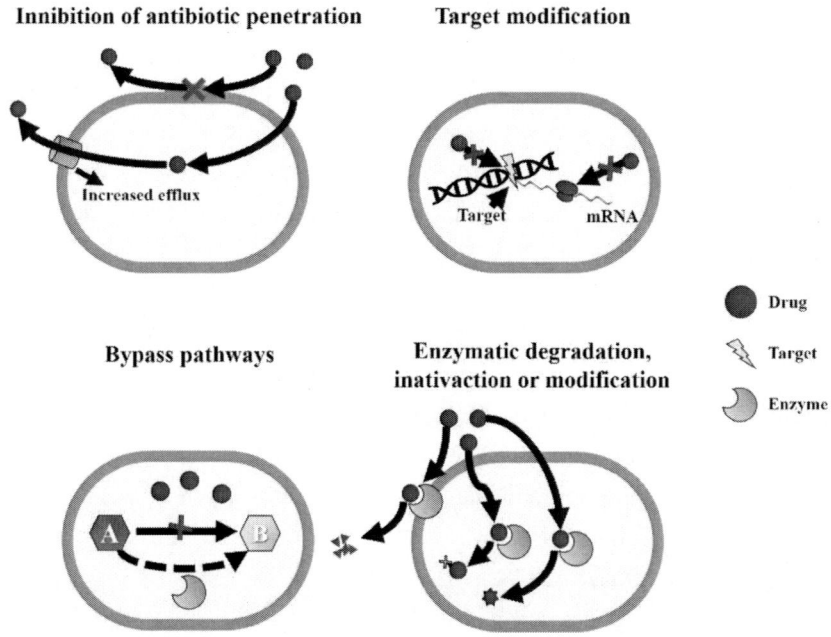

Figure 1. Main mechanisms of antibiotic resistance.

METHICILLIN-RESISTANT *STAPHYLOCOCCUS AUREUS* (MRSA)

History and Infections

The discovery of the bactericidal effects of penicillin isolated from the fungus *Penicillium notatum* by Alexander Fleming in 1928 against *S. aureus* led to mass production of the antibiotic (Fleming, 1929; Neushul, 1993).

However, the industrial production of penicillin was carried out only in 1940 by Howard Florey and Ernst Chain (Fleming, 1945; Durand; Raoult; Dubourg, 2019). Before the discovery of penicillin and its efficacy in the treatment of infections caused by *S. aureus*, the mortality rate of systemic infections caused by this microorganism was about 80% (Skinner; Keefer, 1941; Lowy, 2003).

The discovery of antibiotics allowed the decrease in the mortality rate of patients in hospital units, and soldiers affected by pneumonia and meningitis during World War II (Lewis, 2013). However, large-scale use allowed the appearance of resistant strains in just two years of penicillin use (Rammelkamp; Maxon, 1942; Kirby, 1944). Studies have pointed that at the end of the 1960s, more than 80% of the clinical isolates of *S. aureus* acquired in the community and the hospital field had a resistance profile (Chambers, 2001; Lowy, 2003).

The outbreaks initially occurred in hospital environments, gradually spreading to the community (Hassall; Rountree, 1959). This dissemination lasted approximately 10 years (Jessen et al., 1969). After this period, a decrease in the strain fago 80/81 was observed, which was among those responsible for causing epidemics at the time, which allowed methicillin to be commercially available as an alternative treatment (Rountree; Freeman, 1955; Jessen et al., 1969).

Methicillin began to be applied in the clinic in 1959, and it was the first β-lactamase resistant semisynthetic penicillin. This enzyme is capable of hydrolyzing the β-lactamic ring of the antibiotic being able to inactivate its action (Barber, 1961; Kesharwani; Mishra, 2019). This plasmid-encoded enzyme is transferred by transduction or conjugation, and this mechanism gives the microorganism the resistance to methicillin and is then called methicillin-resistant *Staphylococcus aureus* (MRSA), which is currently found in more than 95% of *S. aureus* worldwide (Lowy, 2003; Bonomo, 2017).

Methicillin-resistant strains were first reported in 1961 in the United Kingdom, and their resistance occurred through the incorporation of the *mecA* gene into the chromosome (Jevons, 1961; Junie et al., 2018). *MecA* encodes an alternative penicillin binding-protein (PBP2a) essential for biosynthesis of the cell wall. The resistance conferred by the *mecA* is broad-spectrum, providing resistance to the entire class of lactate drugs, except ceftaroline and ceftobiprole (Ballhausen et al., 2014; Boswihi; Udo, 2018).

MRSA outbreaks began to be reported globally during the 1980s and 1990s in countries such as the United Kingdom, Ireland, Australia, the Far East and the United States (Thompson; Cabezudo; Wenzel, 1982; Bradley et al., 1985; Faoagali; Thong; Grant, 1992). From this, the infections caused by MRSA were recognized as a global risk, especially for immunocompromised patients generating a considerable problem for the services responsible for the control of these infections (Durand; Raoult; Dubourg, 2019).

These studies show the international and intercontinental dissemination capacity of MRSA, reaching extremely alarming infection percentages. This may be tied to the fact that MRSA infections have been restricted only in hospitals and health facilities, however, enter to the community and animals emerged alarmingly, increasingly identifying outbreaks of MRSA (Hiramatsu et al., 2014; Costa-Júnior et al., 2019; Durand; Raoult; Dubourg, 2019).

When MRSA strains occurred for the first time, they were identified in the elderly, admitted to health institutions, who had a history of previous use of antibiotics. These strains were classified as MRSA associated with health services (HA-MRSA). Over time, MRSA strains were isolated from apparently healthy individuals in the communities and who did not present the previous contact with strains from health institutions. These new MRSA strains were now classified as MRSA strains of community origin (CA-MRSA) (David; Daum, 2010; Junie et al., 2018; Li, 2018).

Clinically the infection caused by CA-MRSA is defined as an infection caused by MRSA diagnosed in an outpatient clinic or within 48 hours of hospitalization if the patient does not present the following risk factors for HA-MRSA: hemodialysis, surgery, residence in an extended stay or hospitalization establishment during the previous year, presence of a permanence catheter or percutaneous device at the time of the patient's past MRSA culture or isolation (Alrabiah et al., 2016; Junie et al., 2018; Li, 2018).

CA-MRSA strains can be differentiated from HA-MRSA strains by their molecular characteristics, in addition to epidemiological characteristics and their spectrum of antibiotic resistance. Subsequently, a new type of MRSA called livestock-associated MRSA (LA-MRSA) was identified (Junie et al., 2018; Li, 2018; Dittmann, 2019). MRSA has also been identified in other animals such as dogs, cats, horses, goats, pigs, and chickens (Pantosti, 2012; Bhattacharyya et al., 2016; Drougka et al., 2016; Da Costa-Junior et al., 2019). Among the strains of LA-MRSA, the most widespread is CC398. Generally, LA-MRSA CC398 exhibits similar potential virulence as *S. aureus* in humans, and it is associated with the same multiple clinical conditions. It can be introduced into hospitals and cause hospital infections, such as postoperative infections at the site of surgery, pneumonia associated with mechanical ventilation, septicemia, and infections after joint replacement. For this reason, it is recommended, for farmers and veterinarians that be in contact with animals, screening for MRSA colonization at hospital admission (Cuny; Wieler; Witte, 2015).

Old Therapeutic Options for MRSA

Treatment for MRSA infections should be guided by local factors, taking into account the sources of infection and risk factors associated with patient populations or the environment, and should be related to updated epidemiological data of local incidence of pathogens and resistant strains (Deresinski, 2007; Luna et al., 2010). Epidemiological data facilitate the choice of antibiotic therapy, associated with an accurate microbiological diagnosis (Luna et al., 2010).

The introduction of resources that aid precise diagnosis and that supports antibiotic therapy is considered a crucial point in the treatment of MRSA infections. The inadequate choice of antibiotics may be associated with increased morbidity and mortality, besides inducing the increase in the resistance rate, evidencing the importance of rational use of these drugs, thus minimizing the selection of resistance to antimicrobials (Kollef et al., 1999; Deresinski, 2007; Baudel et al., 2009).

Vancomycin

Vancomycin is a drug used for more than 50 years for the treatment of MRSA bacteremia (Choo; Chambers, 2016). It is a glycopeptide that acts inhibiting the synthesis of the cell wall. Vancomycin is acting by binding to the D-Ala-D-Ala terminal portion of a pentapeptide found in peptidoglycan precursors, thereby interfering with the transpeptidation step and limiting the strong connection D-Ala- D-Ala with the pentapeptide, hiding it from the transpeptidase that catalyzes cross-link synthesis, leading to destabilization of the cell wall (Table 1) (Kang; Park, 2015).

Although it is associated with benefits in therapy, much is discussed about the best way to use vancomycin (Choo; Chambers, 2016). Studies indicate that inappropriate administration of vancomycin may compromise its pharmacokinetic and pharmacodynamic profile, being associated with an increased risk of failure to treat MRSA infections. The use of individualizing dose, based on the patient's weight, can avoid possible dosage errors and assist in treatment with vancomycin (Kalil et al., 2014; Choo; Chambers, 2016).

The prevalence of MRSA infections spreads in hospitals led to an increase in vancomycin use, which culminated in the development of vancomycin-resistant strains (Luna et al., 2010). Researchers, in 1996, found the first strains with intermediate resistance to vancomycin (VISA), and today the existence of strains with full resistance to vancomycin (VRSA) (Hiramatsu et al., 1997; Luna et al., 2010). The vancomycin resistance mechanism occurs due to the alteration of the D-Ala-D-Ala complex by the *van* gene, replacing the terminal amino acid D-Ala with D-lactate encoded by the *vanA*, *vanB* and *vanD* genes, and replaced by D-serine when encoded by the *vanC*, *vanE* and *vanG* genes and thereby decreasing the affinity of vancomycin with the peptideoglycan layer (Kang; Park, 2015).

Table 1. Antimicrobials used in MRSA infections.

Drug	Molecular formula	Mechanism of action	Spectrum of activity	Treatment	Advantages	Limitations	Reference
Vancomycin	$C_{66}H_{75}Cl_2N_9O_{24}$	Acts on the cell wall by binding to the D-Ala-D-Ala terminal portion of a pentapeptide	Gram-positive bacteria	1000 mg IV 6-6 hour	Effective for various infections caused by *Streptococcus*, *Enterococcus* and *Staphylococcus aureus*.	Low tissue penetration, particularly in the lung, relatively slow bacterial death and toxic potential. Cases of vancomycin-resistant bacteria.	Choo; Chambers, 2016; Chan et al., 2018; Monteiro et al., 2018
Daptomycin	$C_{72}H_{101}N_{17}O_{26}$	Causes rapid depolarization of the cell membrane due to calcium-dependent potassium efflux	Gram-positive bacteria	IV 24-24 hour	Safe and effective for the treatment of several diseases as bacteremia, infective endocarditis on the right and left, osteomyelitis, among others.	Pulmonary surfactant inactivates daptomycin. It should not be used to treat pneumonia. Not recommended for pediatric patients under one year due to likely effects on the muscular, neuromuscular and/or nervous systems.	Gonzalez-Ruiz; Seaton; Hamed, 2016; Taylor; Palmer, 2016; Ye et al., 2019
Oxazolidinone	$C_3H_5NO_2$	Inhibits protein synthesis by binding in the 50S ribosomal subunit.	Gram-positive, gram negative and anaerobic pathogens	600 mg IV or Oral 12-12 hours	Active against a broad spectrum of Gram-positive bacteria, including methicillin and vancomycin-resistant *Staphylococcus*, vancomycin-resistant *Enterococcus*, penicillin-resistant *Pneumococcus* and anaerobes.	High cost and complex procurement method.	Manfredi; Sabbatani, 2010; Cattaneo; Alffenaar; Neely, 2016; Roger; Roberts; Muller, 2018

Drug	Molecular formula	Mechanism of action	Spectrum of activity	Treatment	Advantages	Limitations	Reference
Teicoplanin	$C_{72}H_{68}Cl_2N_8O_{28}$	Inhibits the polymerization of peptidoglycan, resulting in inhibition of bacterial cell wall synthesis, and cell death.	Aerobic and anaerobic Gram-positive bacteria	IV 12-12 hours for 1-4 days	Fewer side effects compared to other antibiotics.	Hypersensitivity reactions (manifesting as hives, fever and stiffness) and gastrointestinal side effects, such as vomiting and diarrhea. Unusual haematological sequelae include eosinophilia, thrombocytopenia and, more rarely, leukopenia.	Khamesipour et al., 2015; Xu et al., 2018; Sarkar; Haldar, 2019

Despite this, the use of vancomycin has not been discontinued, and some studies prove efficacy in the use of vancomycin associated with other antibiotic agents (Damasco et al., 2019). Vancomycin is of great importance in therapy, as it is one of the leading choices in the treatment of resistant β-lactamase infections (Kang; Park, 2015).

Oxazolidinone

With the emergence of vancomycin-resistant strains, the need for new drugs in MRSA therapy allowed the introduction of the class of oxazolidinones (Bozdogan; Appelbaum, 2004; Watkins; Lemonovich; Feli-JR, 2012). Oxazolidinones are 5-member cyclic compounds consisting of a nitrogen atom, an oxygen atom, and a carbonyl group (Table 1). It is a class of synthetic antibacterials active against gram-positive pathogens of multiple resistance, including MRSA, penicillin-resistant streptococci, and vancomycin-resistant enterococci (Pandit; Singla; Shrivastava, 2012). The first drug of this class was linezolid, demonstrating to be effective in a wide range of gram-positive infections, being a fully synthetic compound (Bozdogan; Appelbaum, 2004; Kaiser et al., 2007; Watkins; Lemonovich; Feli-JR, 2012).

Although several oxazolidinones have already been synthesized, such as DuP 7221, DuP 105, eperezoli, among others, the toxicity profiles of some, as well as a low activity when compared to linezolid, made it the primary drug of the classes of the oxazolidinones (Kaiser et al., 2007).

Linezolid presents as a mechanism of action the inhibition of bacterial protein synthesis due to binding to rRNA 23S in the ribosome 50S. It is indicated for the treatment of several conditions, including infections by vancomycin-resistant *Enterococcus faecium* (VRE), nosocomial pneumonia caused by *S. aureus*, among others (Bozdogan; Appelbaum, 2004; Kaiser et al., 2007; Watkins; Lemonovich; Feli-JR, 2012).

Resistance to other protein synthesis inhibitors does not affect oxazolidinone activity. However, it has been reported that the rare development of oxazolidinone resistance cases, associated with changes in 23S r-RNA during treatment (Pandit; Singla; Shrivastava, 2012).

Daptomycin

Daptomycin is classified as a cyclic lipopeptide that acts, preferably in gram-positive bacteria, binding on the membrane of these bacteria and causing rapid membrane depolarization, leading to bacterial cell death (Table 1). The mechanism of action of daptomycin involves the calcium-dependent insertion of the compound in the bacterial cytoplasmic membrane. This bactericidal effect makes daptomycin a useful antibiotic in the treatment of MRSA infections, such as skin and soft tissue infections, endocarditis, and bacteremia (Luna et al., 2010; Gonzalez-Ruiz; Seaton; Hamed, 2016).

Despite the promising therapeutic effects, it has as a limitation its route of administration that should be intravenously only. Even with this limitation, daptomycin is often used for MRSA infections with vancomycin resistance (Luna et al., 2010; Damasco et al., 2019).

In addition to these applications, studies indicate the use of daptomycin in bone and joint infections, also considering the combination of antimicrobials, such as rifampicin or quinolone, against infections caused by *Staphylococcus*, to exert anti-biofilm activity or even prevent the possible appearance of resistance (Telles; Cieslinski; Tuon, 2019).

Although clinical results demonstrate good daptomycin activity against MRSA infections, bacteremia caused by MRSA remains a challenge. Studies indicate that to increase activity and prevent resistance, high doses of daptomycin must be used concomitantly with other antimicrobial agents, which is recommended for the treatment of serious infections (Gonzalez-Ruiz; Seaton; Hamed, 2016).

Although there are reports of resistance to daptomycin, it is still uncommon to find cases of resistance to this drug, thus showing that daptomycin, when associated with other antibiotics, can lead to the resolution of several complex gram-positive infections, in addition to playing an essential role in decreased bacterial resistance (Gonzalez-Ruiz; Seaton; Hamed, 2016).

Teicoplanin

Teicoplanin is a glycopeptide antibiotic used in infections caused by aerobic and anaerobic gram-positive bacteria. Its advantage is the possibility of intramuscular and intravenous administration, is recommended as an alternative to vancomycin and linezolid in MRSA pneumonia, according to the British Thoracic Society (Mukhopadhyay, 2014; Armenia et al., 2018).

Teicoplanin acts by inhibiting the growth of susceptible organisms, acting in cell wall biosynthesis in another region than those affected by beta-lactams (Table 1). It is a complex molecule with a peptide nucleus of seven aromatic amino acids, forming five hydrogen bonds with the terminal d-alanyl-d-alanine of the bacterial cell wall, blocking its synthesis and consequently causing cell lysis (Armenia et al., 2018).

Teicoplanin shows increased potency when compared to vancomycin, particularly against some resistant clinical isolates belonging to the genera *Staphylococcus*, *Streptococcus,* and *Enterococcus*. Therefore, teicoplanin is considered as a last resort for the treatment of severe infections by multiresistant gram-positive pathogens (Armenia et al., 2018).

Although teicoplanin is a drug of choice in the treatment of joint infections caused by *Staphylococcus*, efficacy, safety, and pharmacokinetic data are scarce. Peeters and coworkers (2016) evidenced that teicoplanin can be used as an alternative to replace vancomycin in patients with MRSA infections or with intolerance to beta-lactam antibiotics.

Combined Therapy

Although monotherapy has been used for more than fifty years with the use of vancomycin initially and later with the emergence of new drugs, giving support for severe MRSA infections, the results of MRSA infections present high mortality rates and treatment failure. Clinical studies also show the use of monotherapy, reserving combination therapy for cases where monotherapy has a higher risk of failure (Holland; Davis, 2019).

Daptomycin combined with β-lactams prevents the emergence of resistance to daptomycin in clinical MRSA isolates and *Enterococcus* (Nadrah; Strle, 2011; Berti et al., 2012; Mehta et al., 2012). Daptomycin has also been used in combination with rifampicin, linezolid, phosphomycin, tigecycline, among others in MRSA infections (Gonzalez-Ruiz; Seaton; Hamed, 2016).

Studies have also evaluated the association of daptomycin with ceftaroline, showing that ceftaroline overcomes MRSA resistance to daptomycin, thereby increasing the binding of daptomycin to the cell membrane due to changes in membrane fluidity and load (Barber et al., 2014; Sakoulas et al., 2014).

Dilworth and coworkers (2018) evaluated the benefits of combining vancomycin with phthalactamics, evidencing that the combination accelerates the elimination of MRSA bacteremia compared to vancomycin alone.

Combination therapy presents itself as a viable alternative for the treatment of multidrug-resistant infections and the development of toxicity due to combination therapy sometimes limits its use in the clinic. The development or discovery of new therapeutic options may be an alternative, as well as the encapsulation of drugs into controlled-release nanocarriers, seeking to reduce the toxicity of conventional drugs, as well as improved their therapeutic effect (Holland; Davis, 2019; Lin et al., 2019).

Because most antibiotics have limited efficacy against infections caused by *S. aureus*, new strategies are being implemented, which offer greater therapeutic potential (Zimmerli, 2014; Ansari et al., 2019; Labruère; Sona; Turos, 2019).

NEW THERAPEUTIC APPROACHES FOR MRSA

Natural Products

The discovery of new antimicrobial agents of natural origin is still considered a global challenge. In this sense, current products have been a valuable source of potential antimicrobials for the pharmaceutical industry (Genilloud, 2019). Plants present different levels of defense against microorganisms, such as constitutive chemical defense, direct inducible chemical defense, and gene-inducing chemical defense. These mechanisms produce a variety of secondary metabolites (Abreu et al., 2017).

For this reason, studies look for plants that can potentiate the effects of known antibiotics. Natural products can present promising results and new strategies for treatment in infections caused by MRSA. Aelenei and coworkers (2019) evaluated the antibacterial activity of the extract of the *Morus alba* leaf. Despite moderate antibacterial activity against MRSA ATCC 33591 and ATCC 43300, MSSA ATCC 6538 and *S. epidermidis* ATCC 12228, *Morus alba* leaf extract reversed resistance of MRSA ATCC 43300 to oxacillin. Besides, the extract showed synergy with gentamycin, oxacillin, and tetracycline against all the strains used in this study. These results are significant and suggested *Morus alba* extract as an alternative for the development of new treatment strategies in infections caused by MRSA and *S. epidermidis*.

Another study with promising results was the one carried out by de Souza Constantino and coworkers (2018). The authors evaluated the antimicrobial activity of fractionation products (TSH fraction, halistanol sulfate (HS) and halistanol sulfate C (HS-C)) of the marine sponge *Petromica citrina* against twenty bacteria and two fungi. After initial *in vitro* tests, the *in vivo* trial was proposed to evaluate survival and inflammatory parameters in an animal model of MRSA-mediated peritonitis. The BF fraction, TSH, HS and SH-C were able to inhibit *Enterococcus faecalis*, *S. aureus* and *Candida albicans in vitro*. In general, anti-inflammatory activity was detected in animals treated with TSH in different doses. These data suggest that TSH may be an exciting alternative to treating Gram-positive resistant bacteria infections due to its antimicrobial profile associated with its anti-inflammatory properties.

Hoare and coworkers (2019) analyzed the antimicrobial activity of the extracts of edible Irish algae *Fucus serratus* and *Fucus vesiculosus* against 28 MRSA clinical isolates, including a glycopeptide-intermediate *S. aureus* (GISA) isolate and two strains of *S. aureus* containing the *mecC* gene. The aqueous extract of *F. vesiculosus* was the most promising extract for the prevention and elimination of the biofilm. The results showed that the extracts have a wide variety of antimicrobial activity against the tested strains, with *Fucus vesiculosus* aqueous extract being the most promising. This extract also demonstrated to prevent and discontinue MRSA biofilms, indicating potential as a new antimicrobial and increasing the possibility of its possible use in therapy.

Jiang and coworkers (2017) evaluated myoliolipid (MCL), which presented anti-inflammatory activity in *S. aureus* and MRSA-induced peritonitis. MCL inhibited the expression of inflammatory cytokines and chemokines in macrophages and dendritic cells after stimulation with peptidoglycan, the main composition of the cell wall of gram-positive bacteria. Also, MCL was able to reduce IL-6 secretion by negative regulation of NF-κB activation and improved survival status in mice with a lethal dose of *S. aureus*. Using a mouse model with MRSA infection, MCL dysregulated the expression of IL-6, TNF-α, MCP-1/CCL2, and IFN-γ in serums and increase damage to liver and kidney organs. The researchers concluded that MCL maintains immune balance and decreases the inflammatory response triggered by peptidoglycan, *S. aureus*, and MRSA, thus demonstrating its potential use in sepsis caused by gram-positive bacteria and antibiotic-resistant bacteria, such as MRSA.

Shamsuddin and Basri (2018) evaluated the antibacterial activity of *Canarium odontophyllum* leaf acetone extract against MRSA ATCC 33591 and VISA ATCC 700699 (Mu50 strains). This extract exhibits both bacteriostatic and bactericidal activity against both MRSA strains. Kanga and coworkers (2018) proved that *Albizia lebbeckstem* bark ethanol extract has bacteriostatic and bactericidal activity against multidrug-resistant MRSA strains.

Zhao and coworkers (2019) evaluated the antimicrobial action of Rhodomyrtosone B (RDSB), a natural acyfloroglucinol, isolated from *Rhodomyrtus tomentosa* leaves, against bacteria *in vitro* and *in vivo* studies. RdSB exhibited distinct antibacterial activities against selected gram-positive pathogens responsible for severe infections, such as MRSA and VRE. It is essential to highlight that RdSB showed much faster bactericidal activity against MRSA compared to vancomycin.

Sharifi-Rad and coworkers (2016) evaluated the *in vitro* antimicrobial activity of the methanol extract of *Anagallis arvensis* leaves against clinical MRSA isolates. The results showed MICs of 14.5 ± 0.1 µg/mL, demonstrating that the leaf extract of *A. arvensis* has anti-MRSA properties, which corroborate its traditional therapeutic applications.

Abdi and Dego (2019) evaluated the antimicrobial activity of flower, leaf, stem, and root extracts of the herbaceous plant *Persicaria pensylvanica* against *S. aureus*. The MIC of extracts from the flower, leaf, stem, and root were 62.5 µg/mL, 31.25 µg/mL, 7.8 µg/mL and < 46.9 µg/mL, respectively. Moreover, the crude extract of the different parts of *P. pensylvanica* has a bactericidal effect against *S. aureus*.

Given the studies presented, it is possible to notice that new antimicrobial agents derived from natural products are widely studied. Several of these derivatives have potential compared to MRSA is a good option for the development of new anti-MRSA agents. These natural products and their potent derivatives can be valuable tools for a new mode of action that can overcome drug resistance.

Nanotechnology

Nanotechnology is a science that can be applied in a wide variety of areas, including medical products, food, and cosmetics. The products obtained have a nanoscale strip, with at least one dimension in size range of approximately 1 to 100 nm, and may exhibit different chemical or physical properties. These nanocarriers can promote increased bioavailability, reduced dosage, or increased potency of a drug, and decreased toxicity

(FDA, 2014; Alexander et al., 2016). There is currently a wide variety of nanocarriers, including liposomes, solid lipid nanoparticles, nanoemulsions, micelles, polymeric nanoparticles, metal nanoparticles, among others (Figure 2).

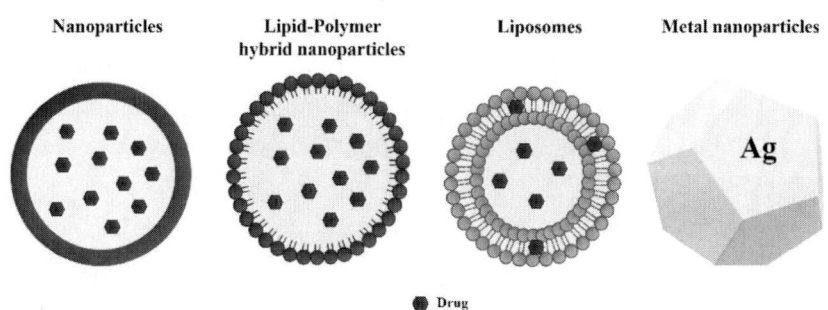

Figure 2. Nanosystems used for MRSA infections.

Polymeric nanoparticles are formed by biodegradable and biocompatible polymers, natural or synthetic, and can be classified into nanocapsules and nanospheres (Yadav et al., 2019). While liposomes are phospholipid vesicles composed of single or multiple concentric lipid bilayers involving aqueous spaces (Mu et al., 2017). The polymeric-lipid hybrid nanoparticles are formed by polymers and lipids. They present characteristics of hydrophobicity and hydrophilicity, conferring a versatile capacity in the encapsulation of several compounds (Mukherjee et al., 2019). Unlike polymeric nanoparticles, metallic nanoparticles are composed of metals, the most commonly used being silver, gold, zinc, copper, sulfur, among other metals (Lee; Jun, 2019).

Li and coworkers (2020) developed a new system of nanoparticles (NP) made from the biocompatible surfactant F-127, tannic acid (TA), and biguanide-based polymetformin (PMET) called FTP NPs. FTP NPs exhibited excellent biocompatibility and could effectively kill *in vitro* MRSA producer of biofilm, with significantly better activity than many peptides or antimicrobial polymers. Also, using the *in vivo* model of a murine wound, FTP NPs achieved a reduction of 1.8 $\log_{10}$ of MRSA bacteria associated with biofilm, which significantly surpassed vancomycin (decrease of 0.8 $\log_{10}$). Thus, FTP NPs presented as a promising approach to MRSA therapy.

Thakur and coworkers (2019) evaluated the combined potential of lipid-polymer hybrid nanoparticles (LPHNs) with fusidic acid (FA) being explored as a promising strategy to combat resistant bacteria in burn infection sites. The potential *in vivo* was also evaluated in the wound model with the bacterium MRSA ATCC 33591 with the determination of parameters such as bacterial load, wound contraction, morphological, and histopathological examination of the wounds. Bacterial count decreased dramatically in the FA-LPHN gel group (FA-LPHN suspension incorporated into Carbopol® 940 (2%, w/v) gel) (5.22 log CFU/mL) on day 3, with significant difference compared to commercial formulation of AF in equivalent concentration (2%, w/w) (FA-CC). The reduction of wound size in the animals treated with FA-LPHN gel (68.70 ± 3.65%) was higher compared to FA-CC groups (73.30 ± 4.23%) and control (83.30 ± 4.40%) on the 5th. This study presented an effective method of formulation for the treatment of MRSA-infected burns, providing a moist environment, and prevention of bacterial infections.

Rukavina and coworkers (2018) analyzed the potential use of different types of liposomes encapsulated azithromycin (AZT) to treat locally skin infections caused by MRSA strains. Conventional liposomes (CLs), deformable liposomes (DLs), liposomes containing propylene glycol (PGLs), and cationic liposomes (CATLs) encapsulated AZT were prepared. All liposomes retained AZT within the skin more efficiently than control and were biocompatible with keratinocytes and fibroblasts. CATLs, DLs and PGLs efficiently inhibited the growth of MRSA strains and were 32 times superior to AZT free in preventing biofilm formation, confirming their potential for topical treatment skin infections caused by MRSA.

A study conducted by Alshamsan and coworkers (2019) evaluated the viability of chitosan-coated liposomes (C-Lips) containing dicloxacillin (DLX) regarding its efficacy against beta-lactam-resistant MRSA strains. DLX-loaded liposomes (DLX-Lips) and chitosan-coated (C-DLX-Lips) demonstrated improved anti-MRSA activity. These results revealed that DLX-Lips and C-DLX-Lips could serve as promising reels for the DLX increasing efficacy against MRSA, which offers a pretty clinical value for the long-term use of DLX.

Bhise and coworkers (2018) proposed the combination of vancomicyn-loaded liposomes (LVAN) and cefazolin-loaded liposomes (LCFZ) for the treatment of MRSA infections. LVAN reduced MIC values 2-fold compared to commercial vancomycin. In turn, treatment with the combination of LVAN and LCFZ showed even more significant results, showing a reduction of 7.9-fold compared to LVAN alone. These results show that formulations developed containing VAN when administered alone or in combination with CFZ provide promising results in combating MRSA infections.

Cavalcanti and coworkers (2018) proposed the association of VAN with usnic acid (UA) and, β-lapachone (β-lap) encapsulated into liposomes (UA-lipo and β-lap-lipo, respectively) as a new therapeutic option against MRSA clinical isolates. The interaction between VAN and β-lap, or liposomes containing β-lap (β-lap-lipo) was synergistic. Additive interaction was found between VAN and UA. UA-lipo resulted in synergism with VAN. Thus, the study demonstrated that VAN in combination with UA-lipo, β-lap or β-lap-lipo, significantly increased its antibacterial activity against MRSA.

Cui and coworkers (2016) evaluated the antibiofilm effect of cinnamon oil encapsulated into liposomes against MRSA. The liposomes improve the chemical stability of the cinnamon oil. As a natural and safe spice, cinnamon oil exhibited satisfactory antibacterial performance in MRSA and its biofilms. The encapsulation of cinnamon oil in liposomes allowed a significant improvement in the time of action of the oil through controlled release, increasing its effectiveness against MRSA and the elimination of biofilms.

Peng and coworkers (2017) developed silver nanoparticles (AgNPs) coated with low molecular weight chitosan (LMWC-AgNPs). The LMWC-AgNPs demonstrated efficacy against MRSA, presenting better biocompatibility and lower body absorption characteristics compared to silver nanoparticles coated with polyvinylpyrrhine (PVP-AgNPs) and silver nanoparticles without surface stabilizer (uncoated AgNPs) in a mouse model with dorsal MRSA wound infection. *In vitro* experiments showed that the three kinds of AgNPs had similar effects to MRSA death. The treatment of mice with MRSA wound infection showed that the three types of AgNPs effectively controlled MRSA wound infection and promoted healing. Thus, the results of this study showed that the LMWC-AgNPs had good anti-MRSA effects, maintaining better biocompatibility and decreasing the body's absorption characteristics.

Goldmann and coworkers (2019) investigated the efficacy of pegylate nanoliposomal formulation encapsulated mupirocin (Nanomupirocin), which was administered parenterally, for the treatment of invasive infections caused by *S. aureus*. The Nanomupirocin exhibited prolonged half-life of active antibiotic and exhibited higher antimicrobial activity against *S. aureus* in comparison to free mupirocin. Nanomupirocin was also more active against MRSA than free mupirocin in a model of neutropenic pulmonary infection of murin. Besides, nanomupirocin was efficiently phagocytized by infected macrophages with *S. aureus*, leading to improve the delivery of mupirocin into the intracellular environment, promoting a more efficient elimination of intracellular staphylococci. The result of this study highlights the potential of nanomupirocin in the treatment of invasive MRSA infections.

New Drug Interaction Studies

In most cases usually, the studies show that synergistic interactions between various metabolites could increase the activity of weak antimicrobial agents. Defense strategies can, therefore, involve the synergistic action of two or more compounds, which can act by different mechanisms and/or targets in the bacteria.

Abreu and coworkers (2017) evaluated the antimicrobial activity of isoflavonoids from *Cytisus striatus*. The researches identified the compounds of plant extracts that could act as antibiotic adjuvants. They showed that isoflavonoids were involved in increasing the antibiotic effect of *C. striatus*. The authors also evaluated 22 other isoflavonoids, from different sources, for their antibacterial and synergistic effects in combination with ciprofloxacin and erythromycin against MRSA strains. It was possible to verify that 22 isoflavonoids enhanced the effect of ciprofloxacin and erythromycin against MRSA strains. The study clearly showed a synergy between isoflavonoids and tested antibiotics, showing its high potential for applications in clinical therapy of antibiotic-resistant microorganism infections, such as MRSA.

The study conducted by Altaf and coworkers (2019) evaluated MRSA susceptibility to various antibiotics associated with non-steroidal anti-inflammatory drugs (NSAIDs). The combination of NSAIDs with antibiotics revealed that meloxicam presented partial synergism with oxytetracycline and gentamycin, while flunixin meglumine showed synergistic effect with oxytetracycline and partial synergism with gentamycin. *In vivo* results revealed that combinations of oxytetracycline with meloxicam/flunixin meglumine and gentamicin with meloxicam/flunixin meglumine were effective. The study concluded that MRSA infections with resistance profiles could be successfully treated by the combination of antibiotics with NSAIDs.

Another study conducted by Alves and coworkers (2019) investigated the responses of the MRSA metabolism when exposed under sublethal concentrations of the synergistic antibacterial combination of nisin + oxacillin. A total of 135 proteins were identified, revealing a change in the expression of 85 proteins after the treatment compared to untreated bacteria. When bacteria were treated using the combination, there was an increase in the expression of resistance-related proteins (e.g., β-lactamase) and also in those involved in protein synthesis, and there was a decrease in protein expression related to stress and changes in proteins related to bacterial energy metabolism. Thus, the changes caused by this treatment affected different proteins related to bacterial biological processes and signaling pathways, such as cell division, structure, regulation, stress, bacterial resistance, gene expression, protein synthesis, energy metabolism, and virulence. These results prove that synergism among antimicrobials has high potential in the therapy and can reduce the need for high amounts of antibacterial substances, besides being useful at different targets in bacterial cells (Alves et al., 2019).

Basri and Sandra (2016) evaluated the interaction of methanol and acetone extract of *Canarium odontophyllum* leaves in combination with oxacillin, vancomycin, and linezolid against MRSA ATCC 33591. The assay revealed that methanol and acetone extracts in association with oxacillin were bactericides, even at subinhibitory concentrations. The results provide evidence that *C. odontophyllum* leaves have the potential to be developed as an antistaphylococcal agent.

Lee and coworkers (2019) investigated the synergistic effect *in vitro* of combined daptomycin-based therapy against 100 MRSA strains. Synergistic effects of daptomycin in combination with phosphomycin, gentamycin, linezolid, oxacillin, or rifampicin against MRSA were useful, including reversing the resistance of several strains to drugs tests. These results demonstrate that the combination of daptomycin with phosphomycin may be an effective therapeutic option for MRSA infection.

Miller and coworkers (2019) reported the interaction *in vitro* of 7.8-didesoxi-griseorodine C of *Streptomyces* sp. with oxacillin against MRSA. The authors proved that the compound is selective against Gram-positive bacteria, including MRSA and *Enterococcus faecium*. Besides, the compound synergizes with oxacillin against MRSA. Simultaneous treatment of the compound with oxacillin resulted in a decrease of approximately ten times in the MIC, indicating synergistic anti-MRSA activity.

In turn, the study conducted by Ma and coworkers (2017) evaluated for the first time the selectively increased antibacterial effects of Bi_2S_3 nanospheres with three classes of ineffective antibiotics, β-lactam (cefuroxime, CXM; cefotaxime, CTX and piperacillin, PIP), a quinolone (ciprofloxacin, CIP), and aminoglycoside against MRSA strains. GEN shows significantly synergistic growth inhibition against MRSA when combined with Bi_2S_3 nanospheres, while CXM, CTX, PIP and CIP do not. Additionally, the combination of Bi_2S_3 and GEN nanospheres can destroy bacterial membrane function and induce more generation of bactericidal reactive oxygen than Bi_2S_3 or GEN alone. This study showed that Bi_2S_3 nanospheres could be used to improve the action of the ineffective GEN antibiotic against MRSA, thus strengthening the antibiotic's ability to combat MRSA infections.

Oh and coworkers (2018) investigated the synergistic antibiofilm effect of the combination of octyl gallate (OG), an antioxidant approved by the U.S. Food and Drug Administration (FDA) as a food additive and bacitracin, with antimicrobial peptide commonly used in antimicrobial ointments. The results of biofilm assays showed that OG allowed bacitracin to inhibit biofilm formation in MRSA. Synergistic antibiofilm activity of bacitracin and OG has also been confirmed in MRSA clinical strains, including USA300, which is the predominant clone of MRSA associated with the community in the USA. This study was the first report on the synergistic antibiofilm activity of an antimicrobial peptide and an antioxidant against MRSA.

Zuo and coworkers (2018) evaluated the anti-MRSA activity of four *Morus alba* root bark prenilflavonoids and their interaction with 11 conventional antibacterial agents. Four prenilflavonoids, i.e., cyclocommunol (Cy), morusinol (Ml), morusin (Mi) and kuwanon E (Ku), were isolated from *Morus alba* bark ethanol extract. Compounds Cy, Mi and Ku showed high antimicrobial activity against *S. aureus* strains susceptible to methicillin (MSSA) and MRSA, including exhibiting bactericidal effect. The compound Ml showed synergy with amikacin (AK) and streptomycin (SM) against all ten MRSA isolates. Ml and Ku also showed synergy with ciprofloxacin (CI), ethycin (EN) and vancomycin (VA) against 7–9 isolates. The study revealed for the first time the anti-MRSA synergism of prenilflavonoids with eleven antibacterial agents and the reversal of MRSA resistance to aminoglycosides, especially amikacin. The results can be valuable for the development of new antibacterial and synergistic drugs against MRSA infection.

Shafiq and coworkers (2017) evaluated two clinical isolates obtained from a 68-year-old male patient with persistent bacteremia by MRSA before and after the development of daptomycin resistance. The pharmacodynamic profile of monotherapies and combinations of cephalothin, daptomycin, cefoxitin, nafcillin and vancomycin was evaluated in pre- and post-daptomycin MRSA isolates. Cefoxitin, nafcillin and vancomycin alone or in combination with ceftaroline failed to generate prolonged bactericidal activity against the post-daptomycin isolate, while a ceftaroline-daptomycin combination resulted in a significant effect. Combinations of daptomycin and ceftaroline are promising against persistent bacteremia by MRSA.

CONCLUSION

Staphylococcus aureus infections are considered the most frequent in the hospital, is one of the leading causes of mortality due to the presence of the most different resistance profiles. In ancient times, the discovery of penicillin was a milestone for medicine, reaching the most diverse forms of manifestations of *S. aureus* infections, being an effective therapeutic alternative. With the emergence of strains resistant to penicillins, concern about the misuse of antibiotics arose, followed by few therapeutic options that could replace the use of penicillins and present the same therapeutic efficacy. Despite the inclusion of new therapeutic classes in the treatment of resistant *S. aureus* strains, it was still not enough due to the emergence of strains resistant to these new therapeutic classes, generating multi-resistant strains. Some studies indicate that combination therapy, with the association of different therapeutic classes, may be a viable alternative in the treatment of multidrug-resistant strains. Another reliable and feasible alternative is the encapsulation of antibiotics in nanocarriers that circumvent the resistance of this microorganism and enhance the therapeutic effect of drugs already widely used. Thus, due to the problematic of the *Staphylococcus aureus* infections, studies on the discovery or development of new therapeutic options need to be continuously carried out.

REFERENCES

Abreu, A. C., Coqueiro, A., Sultan, A. R., Lemmens, N., Kim, H. K., Verpoorte, R., ... & Choi, Y. H. (2017). Looking to nature for a new concept in antimicrobial treatments: Isoflavonoids from *Cytisus striatus* as antibiotic adjuvants against MRSA. *Scientific Reports*, 7(1): 1-16.

Aelenei, P., Luca, S. V., Horhogea, C. E., Rimbu, C. M., Dimitriu, G., Macovei, I., ... & Miron, A. (2019). *Morus alba* leaf extract: Metabolite profiling and interactions with antibiotics against *Staphylococcus* spp. including MRSA. *Phytochemistry Letters*, 31: 217-224.

Alexander, A., Ajazuddin, Patel, R. J., Saraf, S., & Saraf, S. (2016). Recent expandion of pharmaceutical nanotechnologies and targeting strategies in the field of phytopharmaceuticals for the delivery of herbal extracts and bioactives. *Journal of Controlled Release*, 241: 110-124.

Alfouzan, W., Udo, E. E., & Modhaffer, A. (2019). Molecular characterization of Methicillin-resistant *Staphylococcus aureus* in a tertiary care hospital in Kuwait. *Scientific Reports*, 9(1): 1-8.

Alrabiah, K., Al Alola, S., Al Banyan, E., Al Shaalan, M., & Al Johani, S. (2016). Characteristics and risk factors of hospital acquired–methicillin-resistant *Staphylococcus aureus* (HA-MRSA) infection of pediatric patients in a tertiary care hospital in Riyadh, Saudi Arabia. *International Journal of Pediatrics and Adolescent Medicine*, 3(2): 71-77.

Alshamsan, A., Aleanizy, F. S., Badran, M., Alqahtani, F. Y., Alfassam, H., Almalik, A., & Alosaimy, S. (2019). Exploring anti-MRSA activity of chitosan-coated liposomal dicloxacillin. *Journal of Microbiological Methods*, 156: 23-28.

Altaf, M., Ijaz, M., Ghaffar, A., Rehman, A., & Avais, M. (2019). Antibiotic susceptibility profile and synergistic effect of non-steroidal anti-inflammatory drugs on antibacterial activity of resistant antibiotics (Oxytetracycline and Gentamicin) against methicillin resistant *Staphylococcus aureus* (MRSA). *Microbial Pathogenesis*, 137: 103755.

Alves, F. C. B., Albano, M., Andrade, B. F. M. T., Chechi, J. L., Pereira, A. F. M., Furlanetto, A., ... & Fernandes Junior, A. (2019). Comparative proteomics of Methicillin-resistant *Staphylococcus aureus* subjected to synergistic effects of the lantibiotic nisin and Oxacillin. *Microbial Drug Resistance*, 26(3).

Ansari, S., Jha, R. K., Mishra, S. K., Tiwari, B. R., & Asaad, A. M. (2019). Recent advances in *Staphylococcus aureus* infection: focus on vaccine development. *Infection and Drug Resistance*, 12: 1243.

Araújo, R. D. M. P., de Moraes Peixoto, R., Jatobá, L., Peixoto, S., Gouveia, G. V., & da Costa, M. M. (2017). Virulence factors in *Staphylococcus aureus* and quality of raw milk from dairy cows in a semiarid region of Northeastern Brazil. *Acta Scientiae Veterinariae*, 45: 1-8.

Armenia, I., Marcone, G. L., Berini, F., Orlandi, V. T., Pirrone, C., Martegani, E., ... & Marinelli, F. (2018). Magnetic nanoconjugated teicoplanin: a novel tool for bacterial infection site targeting. *Frontiers in Microbiology*, 9: 2270.

Baek, K. T., Gründling, A., Mogensen, R. G., Thøgersen, L., Petersen, A., Paulander, W., & Frees, D. (2014). β-Lactam resistance in methicillin-resistant *Staphylococcus aureus* USA300 is increased by inactivation of the ClpXP protease. *Antimicrobial Agents and Chemotherapy*, 58(8): 4593-4603.

Ballhausen, B., Kriegeskorte, A., Schleimer, N., Peters, G., & Becker, K. (2014). The *mecA* homolog *mecC* confers resistance against β-lactams in *Staphylococcus aureus* irrespective of the genetic strain background. *Antimicrobial Agents and Chemotherapy*, 58(7): 3791-3798.

Barber, M. (1961). Methicillin-resistant staphylococci. *Journal of Clinical Pathology*, 14(4): 385.

Basri, D. F., & Sandra, V. (2016). Synergistic interaction of methanol extract from *Canarium odontophyllum* Miq. Leaf in combination with oxacillin against methicillin-resistant *Staphylococcus aureus* (MRSA) ATCC 33591. *International Journal of Microbiology*, 2016.

Baudel, J. L., Tankovic, J., Carrat, F., Vigneau, C., Maury, E., Lalande, V., ... & Offenstadt, G. (2009). Does nonadherence to local recommendations for empirical antibiotic therapy on admission to the intensive care unit have an impact on in-hospital mortality?. *Therapeutics and Clinical Risk Management*, 5: 491.

Bes, T. M., Martins, R. R., Perdigão, L., Mongelos, D., Moreno, L., Moreno, A., ... & Levin, A. S. (2018). Prevalence of methicillin-resistant *Staphylococcus aureus* colonization in individuals from the community in the city of Sao Paulo, Brazil. *Revista do Instituto de Medicina Tropical de São Paulo*, 60. [*Magazine of the Institute of Tropical Medicine of São Paulo*]

Bhattacharya, M., Wozniak, D. J., Stoodley, P., & Hall-Stoodley, L. (2015). Prevention and treatment of *Staphylococcus aureus* biofilms. *Expert Review of Anti-infective Therapy*, 13(12): 1499-1516.

Bhattacharyya, D., Banerjee, J., Bandyopadhyay, S., Mondal, B., Nanda, P. K., Samanta, I., ... & Bandyopadhyay, S. (2016). First report on vancomycin-resistant *Staphylococcus aureus* in bovine and caprine milk. *Microbial Drug Resistance*, 22(8): 675-681.

Bhise, K., Sau, S., Kebriaei, R., Rice, S. A., Stamper, K. C., Alsaab, H. O., ... & Iyer, A. K. (2018). Combination of vancomycin and cefazolin lipid nanoparticles for overcoming antibiotic resistance of MRSA. *Materials*, 11(7): 1245.

Bonomo, R. A. (2017). β-Lactamases: a focus on current challenges. *Cold Spring Harbor Perspectives in Medicine*, 7(1): a025239.

Boswihi, S. S., & Udo, E. E. (2018). Methicillin-resistant *Staphylococcus aureus*: An update on the epidemiology, treatment options and infection control. *Current Medicine Research and Practice*, 8(1): 18-24.

Bozdogan, B., & Appelbaum, P. C. (2004). Oxazolidinones: activity, mode of action, and mechanism of resistance. *International Journal of Antimicrobial Agents*, 23(2): 113-119.

Bradley, J., Noone, P., Townsend, D., & Grubb, W. (1985). Methicillin-resistant *Staphylococcus aureus* in a London hospital. *Lancet (British edition)*, (8444): 1493-1495.

Cadena, J., Thinwa, J., Walter, E. A., & Frei, C. R. (2016). Risk factors for the development of active methicillin-resistant *Staphylococcus aureus* (MRSA) infection in patients colonized with MRSA at hospital admission. *American Journal of Infection Control*, 44(12): 1617-1621.

Cattaneo, D., Alffenaar, J. W., & Neely, M. (2016). Drug monitoring and individual dose optimization of antimicrobial drugs: oxazolidinones. *Expert Opinion on Drug Metabolism & Toxicology*, 12(5): 533-544.

Cavalcanti, I. M. F., Menezes, T. G. C., Campos, L. A. D. A., Ferraz, M. S., Maciel, M. A. V., Caetano, M. N. P., & Santos-Magalhães, N. S. (2018). Interaction study between vancomycin and liposomes containing natural compounds against Methicillin-resistant *Staphylococcus aureus* clinical isolates. *Brazilian Journal of Pharmaceutical Sciences*, 54(2).

Chambers, H. F. (2001). The changing epidemiology of *Staphylococcus aureus?*. *Emerging Infectious Diseases*, 7(2): 178.

Chan, J. O. S., Baysari, M. T., Carland, J. E., Sandaradura, I., Moran, M., & Day, R. O. (2018). Barriers and facilitators of appropriate vancomycin use: prescribing context is key. *European Journal of Clinical Pharmacology*, 74(11): 1523-1529.

Choo, E. J., & Chambers, H. F. (2016). Treatment of methicillin-resistant *Staphylococcus aureus* bacteremia. *Infection & Chemotherapy*, 48(4): 267-273.

Costa, G. A., Rossatto, F. C., Medeiros, A. W., Correa, A. P. F., Brandelli, A., Frazzon, A. P. G., & MOTTA, A. D. S. (2018). Evaluation antibacterial and antibiofilm activity of the antimicrobial peptide P34 against *Staphylococcus aureus* and *Enterococcus faecalis*. *Anais da Academia Brasileira de Ciências*, 90(1): 73-84.

Cui, H., Li, W., Li, C., Vittayapadung, S., & Lin, L. (2016). Liposome containing cinnamon oil with antibacterial activity against methicillin-resistant *Staphylococcus aureus* biofilm. *Biofouling*, 32(2): 215-225.

Costa-Junior, S. D., da Silva, F. A., & Brandão, S. (2019). Infections caused by Methicillin-resistant *Staphylococcus aureus* (MRSA) and Vancomycin-resistant *Staphylococcus aureus* (VRSA) in Domestic Animals.

Damasco, A. P., Costa, T. M. D., Morgado, P. G. M., Guimarães, L. C., Cavalcante, F. S., Nouér, S. A., & Santos, K. R. N. D. (2019). Daptomycin and vancomycin non-susceptible methicillin-resistant *Staphylococcus aureus* clonal lineages from bloodstream infection in a Brazilian teaching hospital. *Brazilian Journal of Infectious Diseases*, 23(2): 139-142.

David, M. Z., & Daum, R. S. (2010). Community-associated methicillin-resistant *Staphylococcus aureus*: epidemiology and clinical consequences of an emerging epidemic. *Clinical Microbiology Reviews*, 23(3): 616-687.

Deresinski, S. (2007). Principles of antibiotic therapy in severe infections: optimizing the therapeutic approach by use of laboratory and clinical data. *Clinical Infectious Diseases*, 45(Supplement_3): S177-S183.

Dilworth, T. J., Casapao, A. M., Ibrahim, O. M., Jacobs, D. M., Bowers, D. R., Beyda, N. D., & Mercier, R. C. (2018, November). 1066. Adjuvant β-Lactam therapy combined with vancomycin for Methicillin-resistant *Staphylococcus aureus* (MRSA) bacteremia: Does β-Lactam class matter?. In *Open Forum Infectious Diseases* (Vol. 5, No. Suppl_1, pp. S319-S319). US: Oxford University Press.

Dittmann, K., Schmidt, T., Müller, G., Cuny, C., Holtfreter, S., Troitzsch, D., ... & Hübner, N. O. (2019). Susceptibility of livestock-associated methicillin-resistant *Staphylococcus aureus* (LA-MRSA) to chlorhexidine digluconate, octenidine dihydrochloride, polyhexanide, PVP-iodine and triclosan in comparison to hospital-acquired MRSA (HA-MRSA) and community-aquired MRSA (CA-MRSA): a standardized comparison. *Antimicrobial Resistance & Infection Control*, 8(1): 122.

Drougka, E., Foka, A., Koutinas, C. K., Jelastopulu, E., Giormezis, N., Farmaki, O., ... & Spiliopoulou, I. (2016). Interspecies spread of *Staphylococcus aureus* clones among companion animals and human close contacts in a veterinary teaching hospital. A cross-sectional study in Greece. *Preventive Veterinary Medicine*, 126: 190-198.

Durand, G. A., Raoult, D., & Dubourg, G. (2019). Antibiotic discovery: History, methods and perspectives. *International Journal of Antimicrobial Agents*, 53(4): 371-382.

Faoagali, J. L., Thong, M. L., & Grant, D. (1992). Ten years' experience with methicillin-resistant *Staphylococcus aureus* in a large Australian hospital. *Journal of Hospital Infection*, 20(2): 113-119.

FDA – Food and Drug Administration. (2014) *Guidance for industry considering whether an FDA-regulated product involves the application of nanotechnology*. U.S. Department of Health and Human Services.

Ferreira, L. M., Nader Filho, A., Oliveira, E. D., Zafalon, L. F., & Souza, V. D. (2006). Variabilidades fenotípica e genotípica de estirpes de *Staphylococcus aureus* isoladas em casos de mastite subclínica bovina. *Ciência Rural*, 36(4): 1228-1234. [Phenotypic and genotypic variability of Staphylococcus aureus strains isolated in cases of bovine subclinical mastitis. *Rural Science*]

Fleming, A. (1929). On the antibacterial action of cultures of a penicillium, with special reference to their use in the isolation of *B. influenzae*. *British Journal of Experimental pathology*, 10(3): 226.

Fleming, A. (1945). *Penicillin*. Nobel lecture, December 11, 1945, p 83–93. The Norwegian Nobel Committee, the Norwegian Parliament, Stockholm, Sweden.

Gatadi, S., Gour, J., & Nanduri, S. (2019). Natural Product Derived Promising Anti-MRSA Drug Leads: A Mini-Review. *Bioorganic & Medicinal Chemistry*, 27(17): 3760-3774.

Genilloud, O. (2019). Natural products discovery and potential for new antibiotics. *Current Opinion in Microbiology*, 51, 81-87.

Goldmann, O., Cern, A., Müsken, M., Rohde, M., Weiss, W., Barenholz, Y., & Medina, E. (2019). Liposomal mupirocin holds promise for systemic treatment of invasive *Staphylococcus aureus* infections. *Journal of Controlled Release*, 316: 292-301.

Grunenwald, C. M., Bennett, M. R., & Skaar, E. P. (2019). Nonconventional therapeutics against *Staphylococcus aureus*. *Gram-Positive Pathogens*, 776-789.

Hassall, J. E., & Rountree, P. M. (1959). Staphylococcal septicaemia. *Lancet*, 213-17.

Hiramatsu, K., Hanaki, H., Ino, T., Yabuta, K., Oguri, T., & Tenover, F. C. (1997). Methicillin-resistant *Staphylococcus aureus* clinical strain with reduced vancomycin susceptibility. *The Journal of Antimicrobial Chemotherapy*, 40(1): 135-136.

Hiramatsu, K., Katayama, Y., Matsuo, M., Sasaki, T., Morimoto, Y., Sekiguchi, A., & Baba, T. (2014). Multi-drug-resistant *Staphylococcus aureus* and future chemotherapy. *Journal of Infection and Chemotherapy*, 20(10): 593-601.

Hoare, A. H., Tan, S. P., McLoughlin, P., Mulhare, P., & Hughes, H. (2019). The Screening and Evaluation of *Fucus serratus* and *Fucus vesiculosus* Extracts against Current Strains of MRSA Isolated from a Clinical Hospital Setting. *Scientific Reports*, 9(1): 1-9.

Holland, T. L., & Davis, J. S. (2019). Combination Therapy for MRSA Bacteremia: To β or Not to β?. *Clinical Infectious Diseases*, ciz750.

Horino, T., & Hori, S. (2019). Metastatic infection during *Staphylococcus aureus* bacteremia. *Journal of Infection and Chemotherapy*, 26(2): 162-169.

Jessen, O., Rosendal, K., Bülow, P., Faber, V., & Eriksen, K. R. (1969). Changing staphylococci and staphylococcal infections: a ten-year study of bacteria and cases of bacteremia. *New England Journal of Medicine*, 281(12): 627-635.

Jevons, M. P. (1961). "Celbenin"-resistant staphylococci. *British Medical Journal*, 1(5219): 124.

Jiang, X., Wang, Y., Qin, Y., He, W., Benlahrech, A., Zhang, Q., ... & Zheng, Y. (2017). Micheliolide provides protection of mice against *Staphylococcus aureus* and MRSA infection by down-regulating inflammatory response. *Scientific Reports*, 7: 41964.

Junie, L. M., Jeican, I. I., Matroş, L., & Pandrea, S. L. (2018). Molecular epidemiology of the community-associated methicillin-resistant *Staphylococcus aureus* clones: a synthetic review. *Clujul Medical*, 91(1): 7.

Kaiser, C. R., Cunico, W., Pinheiro, A. C., Oliveira, A. G. D., Peralta, M. A., & Souza, M. D. (2007). Oxazolidinonas: uma nova classe de compostos no combate à tuberculose. *Revista Brasileira de Farmacologia*, 88(2): 83-88.

Kalil, A. C., Van Schooneveld, T. C., Fey, P. D., & Rupp, M. E. (2014). Association between vancomycin minimum inhibitory concentration and mortality among patients with *Staphylococcus aureus* bloodstream infections: a systematic review and meta-analysis. *Jama*, 312(15): 1552-1564.

Kanga, Y., Djeneb, C. A. M. A. R. A., Aubin, K. K., & Noël, Z. G. (2018). screening phytochemical and anti-methicillin resistant (MRSA) activity of 70% ethanolic extract from the stem bark of *Albizia lebbeck* (L.) benth. (*Fabaceae*). *Asian Journal of Pharmaceutical Research and Development*, 6(6): 1-6.

Kao, K. C., Chen, C. B., Hu, H. C., Chang, H. C., Huang, C. C., & Huang, Y. C. (2015). Risk factors of methicillin-resistant *Staphylococcus aureus* infection and correlation with nasal colonization based on molecular genotyping in medical intensive care units: a prospective observational study. *Medicine*, 94(28).

Kesharwani, A. K., & Mishra, J. (2019). Detection of β-lactamase and antibiotic susceptibility of clinical isolates of *Staphylococcus aureus*. *Biocatalysis and Agricultural Biotechnology*, 17: 720-725.

Khamesipour, F., Hashemian, S. M., Tabarsi, P., Velayati, A. A. (2015). A review of teicoplanin used in the prevention and treatment of serious infections caused by gram-positive bacteria and compared its effects with some other antibiotics. *Biomedical Pharmacology Journal*, 8(1): 513-521.

Kim, C. J., Song, K. H., Park, K. H., Kim, M., Choe, P. G., Lee, S. H., ... & Kwak, Y. G. (2019). Impact of antimicrobial treatment duration on outcome of *Staphylococcus aureus* bacteraemia: a cohort study. *Clinical Microbiology and Infection*, 25(6): 723-732.

Kirby, W. M. (1944). Extraction of a highly potent penicillin inactivator from penicillin resistant staphylococci. *Science*, 99(2579): 452-453.

Kollef, M. H., Sherman, G., Ward, S., & Fraser, V. J. (1999). Inadequate antimicrobial treatment of infections: a risk factor for hospital mortality among critically ill patients. *Chest*, 115(2): 462-474.

Lakhundi, S., & Zhang, K. (2018). Methicillin-resistant *Staphylococcus aureus*: molecular characterization, evolution, and epidemiology. *Clinical Microbiology Reviews*, 31(4): e00020-18.

Lee, S. H., & Jun, B. H. (2019). Silver Nanoparticles: Synthesis and application for nanomedicine. *International Journal of Molecular Sciences*, 20(4): 865.

Lee, Y. C., Chen, P. Y., Wang, J. T., & Chang, S. C. (2019). A study on combination of daptomycin with selected antimicrobial agents: *in vitro* synergistic effect of MIC value of 1 mg/L against MRSA strains. *BMC Pharmacology and Toxicology*, 20(1): 25.

Lewis, K. (2013). Platforms for antibiotic discovery. *Nature Reviews Drug Discovery*, 12(5): 371-387.

Li, B., & Webster, T. J. (2018). Bacteria antibiotic resistance: New challenges and opportunities for implant-associated orthopedic infections. *Journal of Orthopaedic Research®*, 36(1): 22-32.

Li, J., Zhong, W., Zhang, K., Wang, D., Hu, J., & Chan-Park, M. B. (2020). Biguanide-derived polymeric nanoparticles kill MRSA biofilm and suppress infection *in vivo*. *ACS Applied Materials & Interfaces*.

Li, Z. (2018). A review of *Staphylococcus aureus* and the emergence of drug-resistant problem. *Advances in Microbiology*, 8(1): 65-76.

Lin, A., Liu, Y., Zhu, X., Chen, X., Liu, J., Zhou, Y., ... & Liu, J. (2019). Bacteria-responsive biomimetic selenium nanosystem for multidrug-resistant bacterial infection detection and inhibition. *ACS Nano*, 13(12): 13965-13984.

Liu, C., Bayer, A., Cosgrove, S. E., Daum, R. S., Fridkin, S. K., Gorwitz, R. J., ... & Rybak, M. J. (2011). Clinical practice guidelines by the infectious diseases society of America for the treatment of Methicillin-resistant *Staphylococcus aureus* infections in adults and children. *Clinical Infectious Diseases*, 52(3): e18-e55.

Lowy, F. D. (2003). Antimicrobial resistance: the example of *Staphylococcus aureus*. *The Journal of Clinical Investigation*, 111(9): 1265-1273.

Luna, C. M., Rodríguez-Noriega, E., Bavestrello, L., & Gotuzzo, E. (2010). Treatment of methicillin-resistant *Staphylococcus aureus* in Latin America. *Brazilian Journal of Infectious Diseases*, 14: 119-127.

Ma, L., Wu, J., Wang, S., Yang, H., Liang, D., & Lu, Z. (2017). Synergistic antibacterial effect of Bi2S3 nanospheres combined with ineffective antibiotic gentamicin against methicillin-resistant *Staphylococcus aureus*. *Journal of Inorganic Biochemistry*, 168: 38-45.

Manfredi, R., Sabbatani, S. (2010). Novel pharmaceutical molecules against emerging resistant gram-positive cocci. *Brazilian Journal of Infectious Diseases*, 14(1), 96-108.

Marton, M. (2016). Staphylococcal toxic shock syndrome caused by an intravaginal product. A Case Report. *The Journal of Critical Care Medicine*, 2(1): 51-55.

Miller, B. W., Torres, J. P., Tun, J. O., Flores, M. S., Forteza, I., Rosenberg, G., ... & Concepcion, G. P. (2020). Synergistic anti-methicillin-resistant *Staphylococcus aureus* (MRSA) activity and absolute stereochemistry of 7, 8-dideoxygriseorhodin C. *The Journal of Antibiotics*, 1-9.

Mishra, A. K., Yadav, P., & Mishra, A. (2016). A systemic review on staphylococcal scalded skin syndrome (SSSS): a rare and critical disease of neonates. *The Open Microbiology Journal*, 10: 150.

Monteiro, J. F., Hahn, S. R., Gonçalves, J., & Fresco, P. (2018). Vancomycin therapeutic drug monitoring and population pharmacokinetic models in special patient subpopulations. *Pharmacology Research & Perspectives*, 6(4): e00420.

Mu, L. M., Ju, R. J., Liu, R., Bu, Y. Z., Zhang, J. Y., Li, X. Q., ... & Lu, W. L. (2017). Dual-functional drug liposomes in treatment of resistant cancers. *Advanced Drug Delivery Reviews*, 115: 46-56.

Mukherjee, A., Waters, A. K., Kalyan, P., Achrol, A. S., Kesari, S., & Yenugonda, V. M. (2019). Lipid–polymer hybrid nanoparticles as a next-generation drug delivery platform: state of the art, emerging technologies, and perspectives. *International Journal of Nanomedicine*, 14: 1937.

Mukhopadhyay, J. (2014). Teicoplanin for treating MRSA pneumonia. *BMJ*, 348: g2317.

Neushul, P. (1993). Science, government and the mass production of penicillin. *Journal of the History of Medicine and Allied Sciences*, 48(4): 371-395.

Oh, E., Bae, J., Kumar, A., Choi, H. J., & Jeon, B. (2018). Antioxidant-based synergistic eradication of methicillin-resistant *Staphylococcus aureus* (MRSA) biofilms with bacitracin. *International Journal of Antimicrobial Agents*, 52(1): 96-99.

Palavecino, E. L. (2020). Clinical, epidemiologic, and laboratory aspects of Methicillin-resistant *Staphylococcus aureus* infections. In *Methicillin-Resistant Staphylococcus aureus (MRSA) Protocols* (pp. 1-28). Humana, New York, NY.

Pantosti, A. (2012). Methicillin-resistant *Staphylococcus aureus* associated with animals and its relevance to human health. *Frontiers in microbiology*, 3: 127.

Peng, Y., Song, C., Yang, C., Guo, Q., & Yao, M. (2017). Low molecular weight chitosan-coated silver nanoparticles are effective for the treatment of MRSA-infected wounds. *International Journal of Nanomedicine*, 12: 295.

Rammelkamp, C. H., & Maxon, T. (1942). Resistance of *Staphylococcus aureus* to the Action of Penicillin. *Proceedings of the Society for Experimental Biology and Medicine*, 51(3): 386-389.

Raygada, J. L., & Levine, D. P. Methicillin-resistant *Staphylococcus aureus*: A growing risk in the hospital and in the community. (2009). *American Health & Drug Benefits*, 2(2): 86-95.

Reddy, P. N., Srirama, K., & Dirisala, V. R. (2017). An update on clinical burden, diagnostic tools, and therapeutic options of *Staphylococcus aureus*. *Infectious Diseases: Research and Treatment*, *10*: 1179916117703999.

Reiss-Mandel, A., Rubin, C., Zayoud, M., Rahav, G., & Regev-Yochay, G. (2018). *Staphylococcus aureus* colonization induces strain-specific suppression of interleukin-17. *Infection and Immunity*, 86(3): e00834-17.

Roger, C., Roberts, J. A., & Muller, L. (2018). Clinical pharmacokinetics and pharmacodynamics of oxazolidinones. *Clinical Pharmacokinetics*, 57(5): 559-575.

Rountree, P. M., & Freeman, B. (1955). Infections caused by a particular phage type of *Staphylococcus aureus*. *Medical Journal of Australia*, 2(5): 157-61.

Rukavina, Z., Klarić, M. Š., Filipović-Grčić, J., Lovrić, J., & Vanić, Ž. (2018). Azithromycin-loaded liposomes for enhanced topical treatment of methicillin-resistant *Staphyloccocus aureus* (MRSA) infections. *International Journal of Pharmaceutics*, 553(1-2): 109-119.

Sales, L. M., & Silva, T. M. (2012). *Staphylococcus aureus* meticilina resistente: um desafio para a saúde pública. *Acta Biomedica Brasiliensia*, 3(1): 1-13. [*Staphylococcus aureus* methicillin resistant: a public health challenge. *Acta Biomedica Brasiliensia*]

Santos, A. L. D., Santos, D. O., Freitas, C. C. D., Ferreira, B. L. A., Afonso, I. F., Rodrigues, C. R., & Castro, H. C. (2007). *Staphylococcus aureus*: visitando uma cepa de importância hospitalar. *Jornal Brasileiro de Patologia e Medicina Laboratorial*, 43(6): 413-423. [Staphylococcus aureus: visiting a strain of hospital importance. *Brazilian Journal of Pathology and Laboratory Medicine*]

Sarkar, P., & Haldar, J. (2019). Glycopeptide antibiotics: mechanism of action and recent developments. *Antibiotic Drug Resistance*, 73-95.

Schmidt, T., Kock, M. M., & Ehlers, M. M. (2017). Molecular characterization of *Staphylococcus aureus* isolated from bovine mastitis and close human contacts in South African dairy herds: genetic diversity and inter-species host transmission. *Frontiers in Microbiology*, 8: 511.

Shafiq, I., Bulman, Z. P., Spitznogle, S. L., Osorio, J. E., Reilly, I. S., Lesse, A. J., ... & Tsuji, B. T. (2017). A combination of ceftaroline and daptomycin has synergistic and bactericidal activity *in vitro* against daptomycin nonsusceptible methicillin-resistant *Staphylococcus aureus* (MRSA). *Infectious Diseases*, 49(5): 410-416.

Shamsuddin, N. A. M., & Basri, D. F. (2018). Anti-methicillin resistant *Staphylococcus aureus* (MRSA) activity of an acetone extract from the leaves of *Canarium odontophyllum* (Miq.). *The Journal of Phytopharmacology*, 7(3): 225-229.

Sharifi-Rad, J., Hoseini-Alfatemi, S. M., Miri, A., Sharifi-Rad, M., Sharifi-Rad, M., Hoseini, M., & Sharifi-Rad, M. (2016). Exploration of phytochemical and antibacterial potentiality of *Anagallis arvensis* L. extract against methicillin-resistant *Staphylococcus aureus* (MRSA). *Biotechnology Journal International*, 10(2): 1-8.

Skinner, D., & Keefer, C. S. (1941). Significance of bacteremia caused by *Staphylococcus aureus*: a study of one hundred and twenty-two cases and a review of the literature concerned with experimental infection in animals. *Archives of Internal Medicine*, 68(5): 851-875.

Souza Constantino, L., da Rosa Guimarães, T., de Oliveira, S. Q., Bianco, É. M., de Souza Pessoa, L. G., Michels, M., ... & Reginatto, F. H. (2018). TSH fraction from *Petromica citrina*: A potential marine natural product for the treatment of sepsis by Methicillin-resistant *Staphylococcus aureus* (MRSA). *Biomedicine & Pharmacotherapy*, 108: 1759-1766.

Taylor, S. D., & Palmer, M. (2016). The action mechanism of daptomycin. *Bioorganic & Medicinal Chemistry*, 24(24): 6253-6268.

Taylor, T. A., & Unakal, C. G. (2019). *Staphylococcus aureus*. In *StatPearls* [Internet]. StatPearls Publishing.

Thakur, K., Sharma, G., Singh, B., Chhibber, S., & Katare, O. P. (2019). Nano-engineered lipid-polymer hybrid nanoparticles of fusidic acid: an investigative study on dermatokinetics profile and MRSA-infected burn wound model. *Drug Delivery and Translational Research*, 9(4): 748-763.

Thompson, R. L., Cabezudo, I., & Wenzel, R. P. (1982). Epidemiology of nosocomial infections caused by methicillin-resistant *Staphylococcus aureus*. *Annals of Internal Medicine*, 97(3): 309-317.

Troeman, D. P. R., Van Hout, D., & Kluytmans, J. A. J. W. (2019). Antimicrobial approaches in the prevention of *Staphylococcus aureus* infections: a review. *Journal of Antimicrobial Chemotherapy*, 74(2): 281-294.

Von Eiff, C., Becker, K., Machka, K., Stammer, H., & Peters, G. (2001). Nasal carriage as a source of *Staphylococcus aureus* bacteremia. *New England Journal of Medicine*, 344(1): 11-16.

Watkins, R. R., Lemonovich, T. L., & File Jr, T. M. (2012). An evidence-based review of linezolid for the treatment of methicillin-resistant *Staphylococcus aureus* (MRSA): place in therapy. *Core evidence*, 7: 131.

Werlang, G. O., Haubert, L., Peter, C. M., & Cardoso, M. (2019). Isolation of *Salmonella Typhimurium, Listeria monocytogenes* and coagulase-positive *Staphylococcus* from salami sold at street fairs in Porto Alegre, Brazil. *Arquivos do Instituto Biológico*, 86: 1-6, e0072019.

Xu, G., Chen, E., Mao, E., Che, Z., & He, J. (2018). Research of optimal dosing regimens and therapeutic drug monitoring for vancomycin by clinical pharmacists: analysis of 7-year data. *Zhonghua wei zhong bing ji jiu yi xue*, 30(7): 640-645.

Yadav, H. K., Almokdad, A. A., Sumia, I. M., & Debe, M. S. (2019). Polymer-based nanomaterials for drug-delivery carriers. In *Nanocarriers for Drug Delivery* (pp. 531-556). Elsevier.

Ye, Y., Xia, Z., Zhang, D., Sheng, Z., Zhang, P., Zhu, H., ... & Liang, S. (2019). Multifunctional pharmaceutical effects of the antibiotic daptomycin. *BioMed Research International*, 2019.

Zhao, L. Y., Liu, H. X., Wang, L., Xu, Z. F., Tan, H. B., & Qiu, S. X. (2019). Rhodomyrtosone B, a membrane-targeting anti-MRSA natural acylgphloroglucinol from *Rhodomyrtus tomentosa*. *Journal of Ethnopharmacology*, 228: 50-57.

Zimmerli, W. (2014). Clinical presentation and treatment of orthopaedic implant-associated infection. *Journal of Internal Medicine*, 276(2): 111-119.

Zuo, G. Y., Yang, C. X., Han, J., Li, Y. Q., & Wang, G. C. (2018). Synergism of prenylflavonoids from *Morus alba* root bark against clinical MRSA isolates. *Phytomedicine*, 39: 93-99.

In: Methicillin-Resistant Staphylococcus ...   ISBN: 978-1-53618-189-0
Editor: Erick Pereira Alves   © 2020 Nova Science Publishers, Inc.

Chapter 3

MRSA INFECTIONS AND TREATMENT: SCOPE FOR OPTIONS

Hariharan Periasamy and Gnanamani Arumugam[*]
Microbiology Division, CSIR-Central Leather Research Institute,
Chennai, Tamil Nadu, India

ABSTRACT

Methicillin-resistant *Staphylococcus aureus* (MRSA) are those *S. aureus* isolates carrying a resistance gene *mecA* in their chromosome. Compared to methicillin-susceptible *S. aureus* isolates, MRSA are dreaded as they are resistant to multiple class of antibiotics and only a limited treatment options exist. The MRSA clones cause diverse range of infections both in community and hospitals. These infections include self-resolving skin infections such as impetigo and life-threatening infections such as bacteremia and pneumonia. The ability of MRSA to establish recalcitrant infections is attributed to expression of battery of virulence factors. Management of community MRSA infections is challenging owing to limited MRSA-active oral antibiotic options. Treating nosocomial MRSA infections is much more challenging due to inadequacies in current therapeutic options and underlying comorbidities

---

[*] Corresponding Author's E-mail: gnanamani3@gmail.com; gnanamani@clri.res.in.

in the patients. In this chapter, an overview of signs, symptoms and treatment options for clinically important MRSA infections is presented.

1. INTRODUCTION

Staphylococcus aureus is a Gram-positive bacterium of high medical importance (Figure 1) owing to its ability to cause diverse range of infections both in community and hospitals. The organism is known for its virulence properties and ability to evade antibiotics through acquired resistance mechanisms. Significant proportions of *S. aureus* isolates carry a *mecA* gene that confers the organisms resistance to methicillin and also nearly all β-lactam antibiotics. These isolates are referred as methicillin-resistant *S. aureus* (MRSA) and such isolates are often multi-drug resistant (MDR). Since the first report of MRSA infections, the pathogen has undergone multiple epidemiological manifestations. Vancomycin had been the gold standard drug for treating hospital MRSA infections. Community MRSA infections are being treated by oral antibiotics such as clindamycin and sulphamethoxazole-trimethoprim. Since 2000, several new anti-MRSA drugs have been approved for clinical use. Much of them are intravenous antibiotics and few have oral options. Despite the availability of multiple antibiotic options today, MRSA infections especially the serious infections such as bacteremia and bone and joint infections remain difficult to treat and associated with significant morbidity and mortality.

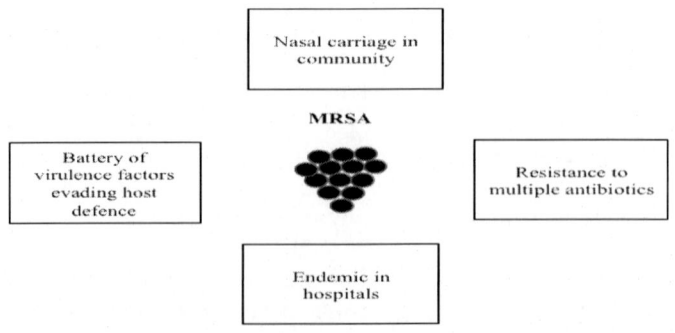

Figure 1. Medical significance of methicillin-resistant *S. aureus*.

2. MOLECULAR BASIS FOR METHICILLIN RESISTANCE

The first MRSA organism was isolated in United Kingdom, almost 60 years back (1961) merely 2 years after the clinical introduction of methicillin (Eriksen 1961). At that time, the predominant β-lactam resistance mechanism in *S. aureus* was penicillinases which are capable of hydrolyzing natural penicillin and also aminopenicillins such as ampicillin and amoxicillin. Methicillin was essentially a discovery to overcome penicillinases which exhibits enzymatic stability to penicillinases. However, MRSA organisms display resistance to methicillin through an acquired penicillin binding protein, PBP2a which is coded by the gene *mecA*. All β-lactams exert their antibacterial action through binding and inactivation of PBPs leading to cessation of cell wall synthesis and cell death. These PBPs play an important role in cell wall synthesis by catalyzing the peptide cross linkage of glycan layers. When *S. aureus* organism carry *mecA* and in the presence of β-lactams, it expresses the PBP2a for which β-lactams show poor affinity. The PBP2a which evades the β-lactams overtakes the functions of β-lactam inactivated PBPs thus cell wall synthesis is not impacted. The *mecA* gene is located on a mobile genomic island referred as staphylococcal cassette chromosome *mec* (*SCCmec*) (Moellering 2012). Based on diversity in genetic makeup, there are 13 distinct *SCCmec* types among the circulating MRSA isolates (Urushibara et al. 2020). The MRSA isolates are largely classified into health care-associated (HA-MRSA) and community-associated (CA-MRSA), depending on their origin. Even at molecular level, there is distinction between HA-MRSA and CA-MRSA clones. The HA-MRSA usually belong to SCCmec I, II and III types and resistant to multiple classes of antibiotics. CA-MRSAs generally belong to SCCmec IV or V types. Unlike HA-MRSA, CA-MRSA are susceptible to many non β-lactam antibiotics (Peng et al. 2018). However, recent reports suggest that CA-MRSAs are increasingly MDR and also entered in to nosocomial settings (Popovich, Weinstein, and Hota 2008).

3. MRSA Infections

S. aureus including MRSA causes diverse infections both in community and hospitals. These are both non-invasive and invasive and the latter are associated with varying degrees of morbidity and mortality depending on the severity of the infections.

4. Skin and Soft Tissue Infections

Skin is the first line of defense against invading bacterial pathogens. Though, diverse bacterial pathogens could able to breach this barrier and set up infections, *S. aureus* is the leading cause of skin and soft tissue infections (Kobayashi, Malachowa, and DeLeo 2015). MRSA causes wide range of skin infections in community, and also in hospitals it is associated with surgical site infections. The community MRSA skin infections are primarily caused by CA-MRSA isolates. The *S. aureus* skin infections are the result of the organism's ability to overcome the defense mounted by neutrophils and macrophages. The organism blocks the chemotaxis of these phagocytic cells and furthermore, it sequesters host antibodies, evades the host immunity through cell wall capsule and bio-film formation (Frank DeLeo 2009). A range of virulence factors are involved in establishing MRSA skin infections. These virulence factors are essentially host cell membrane damaging toxins and bacterial cell wall anchored proteins. The membrane damaging toxins form pores in the host cell cytoplasmic membrane resulting in cell lysis. Bi-component leukocidins, Panton-Valentine leukocidin (PVL), alphahemolysin (alpha-toxin) and phenol-soluble modulins are the important membrane damaging toxins secreted by *S. aureus* (Lacey, Geoghegan, and McLoughlin 2016). The PVL is a two component toxin comprises of LukS-PV and LukF-PV which are secreted individually and assemble in to a pore forming heptamer on neutrophils cell membrane leading to lysis and cell death. The toxin is considered as a strong marker of virulence in community associated MRSA isolates (Shallcross et al. 2013).

4.1. Impetigo

Impetigo is an infection of superficial layers of the epidermis and a common childhood problem. Impetigo has three clinical manifestations *viz.*, impetigo contagiosa, common impetigo, and bullous impetigo. Impetigo contagiosa is the most common childhood infection. The lesion starts with a single 2 – 4 mm erythematous macule which develops in to a vesicle or pustule. These vesicles are easily ruptured leaving an exudate with honey coloured yellow crust over the superficial erosions (Table 1). The skin surfaces exposed to environmental trauma such as nares and perioral regions are often involved. The affected children primarily show skin lesions while mild lymphadenopathy is sometimes present. Most of the times, impetigo contagiosa resolves without the need for treatment. However, in small proportions of children, the condition is complicated with acute glomerulonephritis (Brown et al. 2003).

The bullous impetigo is most frequent in neonates and the infection is exclusively due to *S. aureus*. The lesion is initially large superficial bullae on the trunk and extremities. It can also develop in anogenital region and buttocks of neonates. The encased fluid in the bullae progresses from being clear yellow to turbid and darkish yellow. Within one or two days, the pustules rupture resulting in thin, light brown to golden yellow crusts and a characteristic collarette of scale at the periphery of the lesions (Geria and Schwartz 2010). The bullous form is often the result of infection of intact skin by exfoliative toxin secreting *S. aureus* which is referred as staphylococcal scalded skin syndrome (Darmstadt and Lane 1994).

The common impetigo is also referred as secondary impetigo. The condition can be seen both in children and adults. It is basically the result of secondary impetiginization of conditions that disrupt the integrity of the epidermis, including insect bites, abrasions, varicella, dermatitis, tinea capitis, pediculosis, and scabies. The common impetigo can also complicate systemic diseases such as diabetes mellitus and AIDS. The clinical presentation is similar to that of impetigo contagiosa (Brown et al. 2003; Geria and Schwartz 2010).

In general, impetigo is a self-limiting condition with spontaneous resolution of lesions. Therefore, in the case of uncomplicated infections, observation is an option (Bangert, Levy, and Hebert 2012). Nevertheless, antibiotic treatment is preferred to prevent the complications, expedite the resolution, and also to prevent the relapse. Since, impetigo is more common in children and infants, topical antibiotic treatment is routinely employed. The MRSA active, commonly used topical antibiotics (Table 2) are mupirocin, fusidic acid and nadifloxacin (Geria and Schwartz 2010). Mupirocin which inhibits bacterial protein and RNA synthesis is known for potent activity against MRSA. Clinical studies have shown the effectiveness of mupirocin (2% topical) in the treatment of impetigo (Dagan and Bar-David 1992). Fusidic acid is a steroidal antibiotic that inhibits bacterial elongation factor. The antibiotic exhibits excellent activity against *S. aureus* including MRSA (Fernandes 2016). The utility of fusidic acid (2%) in the treatment of impetigo has been well reported (Koning et al. 2002; Wilkinson 1998; Schofer and Simonsen 2010). Though mupirocin and fusidic acid have been in use for the years in treating MRSA impetigo, the rise in the resistance to these agents is also in reports (Patel, Gorwitz, and Jernigan 2009; Poovelikunnel, Gethin, and Humphreys 2015; Antonov et al. 2015; Dobie and Gray 2004; Brown and Thomas 2002). Nadifloxacin is a fluoroquinolone antibiotic exhibiting activity against MRSA isolates. The topical nadifloxacin (1%) is also an important option for the treatment of impetigo. Various studies have shown the effectiveness of nadifloxacin in treating impetigo (Jacobs and Appelbaum 2006; Narayanan et al. 2014; Nenoff, Haustein, and Hittel 2004). Retapamulin belongs to pleuromutilin class and approved by US FDA for the treatment of bacterial skin infections. Retapamulin is active against MRSA including those resistant to mupirocin and fusidic acid (Woodford et al. 2008). Clinical studies have shown the effectiveness of retapamulin in the treatment of impetigo (Oranje et al. 2007; Koning et al. 2008). Retapamulin is an alternative topical treatment option for the treatment of impetigo caused by mupirocin and or fusidic acid resistant MRSA isolates. When topical treatment is not responsive, systemic antibiotics such as clindamycin and sulphamethoxazole-trimethoprim are preferred (Hartman-Adams, Banvard, and Juckett 2014; Bowen et al. 2017).

However, the clinicians should be aware that some MRSA isolates are resistant to clindamycin or sulphamethoxazole-trimethoprim. Further, on-therapy resistant development is a possibility with clindamycin therapy if the isolate harbours inducible macrolide resistance mechanism (Levin et al. 2005).

Table 1. Clinical manifestations of nonbullous and bullous impetigo

Type of impetigo	Predisposing factor	Characteristic clinical signs
Impetigo contagiosa (Nonbullous impetigo)	Infection of traumatized skin	Small, delicate vesicles or pustules in extremities or face rupture to form honeycolored, crusted plaque
Bullous impetigo	Infection of intact skin	Large, flaccid, transparent vesicles in the face, buttocks, trunk, perineum, and extremities

Table 2. Topical antibiotics active against MRSA

Antibiotic	Formulation	Mechanism of action
Mupirocin	2%	RNA synthetase inhibitor
Fusidic acid	2%	Bacterial elongation factor inhibitor
Nadifloxacin	1%	Topoisomerases inhibitor
Retapumulin	1%	Protein synthesis inhibitor

4.2. Other Skin and Soft Tissue Infections in Community

Apart from impetigo, other community MRSA skin infections are cutaneous abscess, non-purulent and purulent cellulitis, necrotizing fasciitis and deeper infection such as myositis and pyomyositis (Tong et al. 2015). The pyogenic abscess caused by *S. aureus* initiates as local acute inflammatory response to the infection. Recognising the infection, the host mounts a pro-inflammatory response which comprises of release of antimicrobial peptides, accumulation of neutrophils and inflammatory exudate at the site of infection. Therefore, the abscess is made up of viable and dead neutrophils, tissue debris, fibrin, live and dead bacteria (Kobayashi, Malachowa, and DeLeo 2015). Clinically, cutaneous abscess is presented as tender and fluctuant or erythematous with induration (Fitch et al. 2007).

Cellulitis is the result of infection of deep dermis and subcutaneous tissue. Clinically, the condition is presented as an acute, spreading, poorly demarcated area of erythema. The classical inflammatory signs such as pain, redness and swelling are always present. Cellulitis more commonly involves lower extremities and in some instances, upper extremities, abdominal wall, and face are also affected (Raff and Kroshinsky 2016; Tong et al. 2015). The purulent cellulitis is associated with purulent discharge or accumulation of exudate. Clinically, it may be difficult to differentiate purulent cellulitis and cutaneous abscess (Lee et al. 2015).

Necrotizing fasciitis is the fulminant infection of subcutaneous tissue and fascia, mostly in extremities with no involvement of dermis at initial stage. Unlike other community skin infections, necrotizing fasciitis is a serious one and if untreated may result in complications and mortality (Raff and Kroshinsky 2016). There are several case reports showing the involvement of MRSA in necrotizing fasciitis (Lee et al. 2007; Dehority et al. 2006; Lee et al. 2006). MRSA can also cause myositis and pyomyositis which are infection and inflammation of muscle. The treatment of above described infections primarily involves use of oral anti-MRSA drugs. However, complicated cases require hospitalization and intravenous drugs acting on MRSA. The preferred oral antibiotics are clindamycin and sulphamethoxazole-trimethoprim (Khawcharoenporn and Tice 2010).

4.3. Surgical Site Infections

Surgical site infections are those typically causing infections within 30 or 90 days after a surgical operation. The infection involves the incision area and or deeper tissue at the site of surgery. Surgical site infections are classified into incisional and those involving organ and organ space. The incisional infections are further classified into superficial (skin and subcutaneous tissue) and deep (deep soft tissue– muscle and fascia) (Nichols and Florman 2001). In the case of superficial infections, a characteristics purulent discharge is present. Deep incisional infection is found within 30 or 90 days after the operative procedure and involves deep soft tissues of the incision (e.g., fascial and muscle layers). There is a localized pain and tenderness and pyrexia. In case of infections those involving organ and organ space, they occur within 30 or 90 days (for a sub-group of procedures) after the operative procedure and involves any part of the body deeper than the fascial/muscle layers, that is opened or manipulated during the operative procedure (Vera 2017).

The significance of surgical site infection is that it is one of the most common infections in hospitals. Though the etiology of surgical site infections is polymicrobial in nature depending on the common flora present in the patient, *S. aureus* is the leading causative pathogen (Owens and Stoessel 2008; Anderson and Kaye 2009). A published study shows involvement of *S. aureus* in 40.5% cases of surgical site infections. Among the *S. aureus*, 33.8% were MRSA which signifies the role of MRSA in surgical site infections (Weigelt et al. 2010).

Intravenous therapy with anti-MRSA antibiotics combined with other antibiotics that provide coverage of concomitant Gram-negative infections is the common strategy in managing surgical site infections. Since its introduction to clinical practice, the glycopeptide antibiotic vancomycin remained as a gold standard therapy for surgical site MRSA infections. Apart from vancomycin, other antibiotic options are teicoplanin, ceftaroline, daptomycin and linezolid (Weigelt et al. 2004; Eckmann and Dryden 2010).

5. BACTEREMIA

Bacteremia caused by MRSA is one of the therapeutically challenging nosocomial infections. The condition is associated with high mortality and also high treatment cost. Generally, bacteremia is not a primary infection rather secondary manifestation of other invasive infections. The ability of MRSA in successfully expressing virulence factors amidst host defence is the key factor in establishing blood stream infection. The SENTRY surveillance data reveals that globally, *S. aureus* is the second most causative agent in causing blood stream infections (18.7% of blood stream infections). The data also shows that about 33% of *S. aureus* causing bacteremia are MRSA. Several publications show the widespread prevalence of MRSA bacteremia (Cunha, Mikail, and Eisenstein 2008; DeSena, Steele, and Young 2010; Forestier et al. 2007; Hassoun, Linden, and Friedman 2017; Jayaweera et al. 2017; Kempker et al. 2010). Years back, MRSA bacteremia was primarily caused by hospital acquired MRSA clones but in the last 15 years proportion of community associated MRSA has been increasing. For instance, USA300 is the dominant CA-MRSA clone involved in bacteremia.

Medically, *S. aureus* bacteremia is defined as the presence of ≥1 positive blood culture for *S. aureus* in patients with signs and symptoms consistent with an infection. Bacteremia is defined as hospital-acquired if the first positive blood culture was performed more than 48 hours after admission either to the intensive care unit (ICU) or to another hospital ward (Bassetti et al. 2017).

As mentioned earlier *S. aureus* bacteremia is the secondary manifestation of primary infections elsewhere. Catheter related infection (line infections), infective endocarditis, osteoarticular infections (bone and joint infections), skin and skin structure infections, pulmonary infection (pneumonia) are the primary foci of infection (Tong et al. 2015). A bacteremia case can be uncomplicated or complicated. The uncomplicated cases are those show resolution of fever and negative blood culture after the removal of catheter and in response to antibiotic treatment. The complications are often metastatic infections such as infective endocarditis, septic arthritis and osteomyelitis. Furthermore, *S. aureus* bacteremia has the potential to cause life-threatening sepsis. Understanding the difference between uncomplicated and complicated bacteremia is important as management approaches are different. Before the discovery of antibiotics, the mortality due to *S. aureus* bacteremia was >80% and even now it ranges between 15 – 50% (Pastagia et al. 2012; Sit et al. 2018; Yang et al. 2018;

Tong et al. 2015; osé Romero-Vivas 1995). Several patient factors are related mortality due to bacteremia. These are advanced and other comorbidities such as malignancy and renal impairments. Due to therapeutic challenges involved in treating MRSA bacteremia, the disease imposes a huge economic burden.

Intravenous anti-MRSA antibiotics are the corner stone therapy for managing MRSA bacteremia. Identifying the source of infection such as catheter and removing the source is also critical. Infectious disease society of America (IDSA) recommends using either vancomycin or daptomycin as 1st line agent (Liu et al. 2011). Among the two, daptomycin is a strong bactericidal agent, a feature essential for tackling the bacteria in the circulation. Clinical data also suggests a slight edge for daptomycin in managing MRSA bacteremia. The other factor which also does not favour vancomycin is frequent report of nephrotoxicity (Bamgbola 2016). This is particularly problematic in patients who are already suffering from renal impairment. Moreover, recent pharmacokinetic/pharmacodynamic studies revealed the need for higher vancomycin doses mainly to tackle MRSA isolates with slightly higher MICs for vancomycin. In such situations, in order to avoid nephrotoxicity and treatment failure, therapeutic drug monitoring is necessary (Moise et al. 2016; Ye et al. 2016; Ye, Li, and Zhai 2014). Despite all these factors, owing to its decades of use driven clinical experience, vancomycin still remains the mainstay 1st line agent. In order to achieve consistent clinical efficacy, a 24 h-area under the curve (AUC) to minimum inhibitory concentration (MIC) ratio ≥400 is required (Hassoun, Linden, and Friedman 2017). Since, estimating AUC/MIC requires multiple sampling from patients, a trough concentration of 15 -20 mg/L is used as a surrogate marker for an AUC/MIC ratio of ≥400 (Rybak et al. 2009). The duration of therapy depends on whether the bacteremia is uncomplicated or complicated as assessed by clinicians.

Daptomycin is generally reserved for cases in which vancomycin therapy does not show improvement. The IDSA recommends a high dose of daptomycin (8 – 10 mg/kg) for the complicated MRSA bacteremia for better outcome and to prevent resistance development (Liu et al. 2011). The biggest limitation of daptomycin is that the drug is inactivated by lung surfactant. Therefore, daptomycin can't be used for treating bacteremia originated from lung (Silverman et al. 2005).

Table 3. Comparative profile of vancomycin and daptomycin

Property	Vancomycin	Daptomycin
Original source	Streptomyces orientalis	Streptomyces roseosporus
Chemical nature	Glycopeptide	Lipopeptide
Route of administration	Intravenous	Intravenous
Standard dose regimen for adults with normal kidney function	1 g every 12 h	4 mg/kg
Bactericidal activity	Slow	Rapid
Pharmacokinetic/Pharmacodynamic driver	AUC/MIC	AUC/MIC
Concentration maximum, mean (Cmax)	63 mg/L	57.8 mg/L
Half-life, mean	4 – 6 h	8.1 h
Protein binding	55%	90 – 93%
Primary route of elimination	Kidneys	Kidneys
Toxicity	Nephrotoxicity	Myopathy and rhabdomyolysis
Resistance	Vancomycin intermediate sensitive S. aureus (VISA) Vancomycin resistant S. aureus (VRSA)	Cross resistance to VISA

Apart from vancomycin and daptomycin, other agents that can be used as alternatives in treating MRSA bacteremia are telavancin, oritavancin, daptomycin, linezolid, ceftaroline and combination therapies (Ortwine and Bhavan 2018). These agents are useful in cases bacteremia persists (persistent MRSA bacteremia) despite the treatment with 1st line agents. Table 3 depicts comparative profile of vancomycin and daptomycin in detail.

6. PNEUMONIA

The involvement of MRSA in hospital pneumonia is relatively a recent clinical trend. Otherwise, MRSA were found mainly in hospitalized elderly patients and uncommonly in patients in community suffering from pneumonia. However, during the last 20 years, there has been increase in pneumonia caused by MRSA. Presently, MRSA is implicated in 20 - 40% of all hospital acquired bacterial pneumonia and ventilator associated pneumonia. Some of the risk factors of MRSA pneumonia are tobacco use, chronic obstructive pulmonary disease, illicit drug use, previous antibiotic exposure, previous hospitalization, previous history of MRSA infection and viral respiratory tract infections. The clinical signs and symptoms of MRSA pneumonia are indistinguishable from pneumonia causes by Gram- negative pathogens. The classical signs and symptoms are hyperthermia or hypothermia, chills, rigors, cough, purulent sputum production, chest pain, difficulty in breathing and the presence of infiltrated in chest radiograph (American Thoracic and Infectious Diseases Society of 2005). The hospital MRSA infections are commonly present in elderly. Most of the patients suffering from MRSA pneumonia required mechanical ventilation.

Diagnosis of presence of MRSA infections in hospital and community pneumonia cases is challenging. MRSA pneumonia is associated with significant mortality (Rubinstein, Kollef, and Nathwani 2008; Tadros et al. 2013). Aggressive intravenous therapy is necessary for MRSA pneumonia. The challenge is that the antibiotic needs to penetrate the blood-lung barrier to attain adequate concentrations in the lung parenchyma. Though vancomycin has been the 1st line of therapy for MRSA pneumonia, the drug performance is relatively poor compared to that of linezolid. Apart from vancomycin and linezolid, ceftaroline is an option to be regarded but the drug does not have formal approval for MRSA pneumonia. Combination therapies are also often used for better clinical outcome and also to minimize the risk of resistance development (Liu et al. 2011).

7. BONE AND JOINT INFECTIONS

There are three types of osteoarticular infections *viz.*, osteomyelitis, native joint septic arthritis and prosthetic joint infection in which *S. aureus* is the leading causative pathogen.

7.1. Osteomyelitis

Osteomyelitis is an infection of bone resulting in its inflammatory destruction, bone necrosis, and new bone formation. *S. aureus* is identified in 30 – 60% cases of osteomyelitis. There are three types of osteomyelitis; hematogenous osteomyelitis, contagious-focus osteomyelitis and osteomyelitis with vascular insufficiency. Among these three, hematogenous osteomyelitis is more common with the involvement of *S. aureus* which is typically manifested as vertebral osteomyelitis in adults and long bone osteomyelitis in children. Several publications report incidences of MRSA associated osteomyelitis suggesting widespread prevalence of this infection (Tong et al. 2015; Prabhoo et al. 2019).

The virulence factors of *S. aureus* help to establish the bone infections. The organisms express microbial surface components recognizing adhesive matrix molecules (MSCRAMM) which are surface receptors adhere to bone substances, thus colonization is established. Moreover, *S. aureus* possesses the ability to form biofilm in bone environment and evades from host immunity. The antibiotics used to treat bone infections do not reach the site of infection. It has been also reported that *S. aureus* enters osteoblasts and survive inside the cells (Tong et al. 2015; Nair, Williams, and Henderson 2000).

Clinically, the vertebral osteomyelitis is found at the endplates of two adjacent vertebrae and the contacting discs. The route of infection is either through haematogenous or contiguous spread. The disease pathology comprises of severe inflammation, impairment of vasculature, and localized bone loss and destruction.

The primary symptom is back pain in nearly all patients. Fever is another symptom but not consistent among the patients. Nerve compression leading to leg weakness is present in some cases. The complications of infectious osteomyelitis lead to neurologic dysfunctions. Diagnosing the MRSA osteomyelitis is difficult due to two reasons: (i) variable clinical presentation of osteomyelitis; (2) the difficulty in establishing presence of MRSA infection. Various aspects such as patient history, blood cells profile, erythromycin sedimentation rate, level of C-reactive protein, imaging tests (ultrasound, computed tomography, magnetic resonance imaging), microbiological investigation and histopathology are required for the diagnosis (Sheftel et al. 1985; Kavanagh et al. 2018).

The management of MRSA osteomyelitis is very challenging and requires combinations of approaches such as general patient management, prolonged antibiotic therapy and surgical interventions. The debridement of affected area and the surgical necrotic bone or prosthetic material is required for the successful management of infectious osteomyelitis. Since, long term antibiotic treatment is necessary, patients prefer initial intravenous therapy followed by oral antibiotics to avoid hospitalization and minimize the cost. Another important aspect is that the chosen antibiotic has to penetrate from the blood to the site of infection. Furthermore, the antibiotic should able to overcome the biofilm mediated resistance (Kavanagh et al. 2018).

Vancomycin is the drug of choice to initiate the treatment against MRSA osteomyelitis. Teicoplanin (once-daily) is another alternative which can be administered at home or at OPAT centres. But, both agents are poor in penetrating the *S. aureus* biofilm. The current oral options are rifampicin clindamycin, sulphamethaxazole-trimethoprim and linezolid. However, the presence of inducible macrolide resistance mechanism in the infecting MRSA is a risk factor for clindamycin therapy. Though linezolid is highly active against MRSA, it is bacteriostatic and also prolonged therapy leads to myelosuppression. The newly approved delafloxacin (oral) is also active against MRSA, but being a fluoroquinolone, not suitable for pediatric and elderly patients. Rifampicin is an oral drug, known for anti-biofilm activity and also possesses anti-MRSA activity.

Therefore, rifampicin is suitable for treating MRSA osteomyelitis but combined with other antibiotic to prevent resistance development (Spellberg and Lipsky 2012; Kavanagh et al. 2018; Mruk and Record 2012).

7.2. Septic Arthritis

In adults, septic arthritis is predisposed by joint diseases such as rheumatoid arthritis. Moreover, old age (>80 years) is an important predisposing factor for septic arthritis. In children, septic arthritis is a complication of spreading contiguous osteomyelitis. Though, *S. aureus* is the leading causative organism, the proportion of MRSA is lower. Clinically, the condition is primarily manifested as monoarticular infection. Among the various joints, knee is commonly involved and followed by hip and shoulders. The clinical symptoms are single swollen and tender joint with redness and pain. The affected joint becomes immobile due to swelling. In order to confirm the septic arthritis, arthocentesis is performed in which increase in synovial leukocytes count is noted. The presence of *S. aureus* can be confirmed by Gram straining of synovial fluid. Further, the inoculating the synovial fluid in to appropriate culture media helps in isolating the infecting *S. aureus* and determining the methicillin resistance (Tong et al. 2015).

Similar to other bone and joint and infections, treating septic arthritis especially those involving MRSA is therapeutically challenging. Surgical interventions and prolonged antibiotic therapy with combinations of anti-MRSA antibiotics is necessary.

8. INFECTIVE ENDOCARDITIS

This is the one of the serious infection caused by *S. aureus* and associated with high mortality. *S. aureus* is the most common microbial cause of infective endocarditis. Among all infective endocarditis, the proportion of *S. aureus* infection ranges from 15 - 30%. Even those survive from this infection may suffer from complication of embolization of vegetation or metastatic infection. The risk factors for *S. aureus* infective endocarditis are intravenous drug administration, diabetes mellitus, old age, prior cardiac surgery, underlying valvular heart disease, previous endocarditis, presence of intravascular device, persistent bacteremia and male gender (Bamberger 2007).

The cause for the infective endocarditis is the damage to inner endothelium layer in the heart. The damage happens due to either direct trauma (intravascular catheters and electrodes, injected particulate matter from intravenous injection, or turbulent blood flow resulting from valvular abnormalities) or inflammation. The damage to endothelium results in exposure of subendothelial cells which elicits the production of extracellular matrix proteins and tissue factor on which sterile vegetation is formed. If the vegetation is infected with bacteria, it leads to infective endocarditis.

The clinical manifestation of infective endocarditis depends on the involved part of the heart. In case of left-sided endocarditis, dyspnoea and central nervous system symptoms are present. The underlying problems in left-sided endocarditis are heart block, Oslerian manifestations, aortic or mitral valve regurgitation and arterial emboli. In case of right sided endocarditis, dyspnoea, pleuritic chest pain, cough with sputum and haemoptysis are present. The underlying symptoms are tricuspid or pulmonary regurgitation, lung consolidation and effusion.

The treatment of infective endocarditis is highly challenging. Among all anti-MRSA antibiotics, daptomycin is the only drug, evaluated for its effectiveness against infective endocarditis. Aggressive antibiotic therapy with combination of intravenous antibiotics is necessary for treating infective endocarditis (Tong et al. 2015). The overall approved intra-venous anti-MRSA antibiotics, their indications and dose regimens for adults and pediatric patients is summrized in Table 4.

Table 4. Approved intra-venous anti-MRSA antibiotics, their indications and dose regimens for adults and pediatric patients

Drug	Indications	Dose regimens
Vancomycin	Vancomycin is indicated for the treatment of serious or severe infections caused by susceptible strains of methicillin-resistant (beta-lactam-resistant) staphylococci. It is indicated for penicillin-allergic patients, for patients who cannot receive or who have failed to respond to other drugs, including the penicillins or cephalosporins, and for infections caused by vancomycin-susceptible organisms that are resistant to other antimicrobial drugs. Vancomycin is indicated for initial therapy when methicillin-resistant staphylococci are suspected, but after susceptibility data are available, therapy should be adjusted accordingly. Vancomycin is effective in the treatment of staphylococcal endocarditis. Its effectiveness has been documented in other infections due to staphylococci, including septicemia, bone infections, lower respiratory tract infections, skin and skin structure infections. When staphylococcal infections are localized and purulent, antibiotics are used as adjuncts to appropriate surgical measures.	Adults: The usual daily intravenous dose is 2 g divided either as 500 mg every 6 hours or 1 g every 12 hours. Each dose should be administered at no more than 10 mg/min or over a period of at least 60 minutes, whichever is longer. Other patient factors, such as age or obesity, may call for modification of the usual intravenous daily dose. Pediatrics: The usual intravenous dosage of vancomycin is 10 mg/kg per dose given every 6 hours. Each dose should be administered over a period of at least 60 minutes. Close monitoring of serum concentrations of vancomycin may be warranted in these patients.

MRSA Infections and Treatment: Scope for Options

Drug	Indications	Dose regimens
	Vancomycin has been reported to be effective alone or in combination with an aminoglycoside for endocarditis caused by Streptococcus viridans or S. bovis. For endocarditis caused by enterococci (e.g., E. faecalis), vancomycin has been reported to be effective only in combination with an aminoglycoside. Vancomycin has been reported to be effective for the treatment of diphtheroid endocarditis. Vancomycin has been used successfully in combination with either rifampin, an aminoglycoside, or both in early-onset prosthetic valve endocarditis caused by S. epidermidis or diphtheroids. Specimens for bacteriologic cultures should be obtained in order to isolate and identify causative organisms and to determine their susceptibilities to vancomycin. To reduce the development of drug-resistant bacteria and maintain the effectiveness of vancomycin and other antibacterial drugs, vancomycin should be used only to treat or prevent infections that are proven or strongly suspected to be caused by susceptible bacteria. When culture and susceptibility information are available, they should be considered in selecting or modifying antibacterial therapy. In the absence of such data, local epidemiology and susceptibility patterns may contribute to the empiric selection of therapy.	

Table 4. (Continued)

Drug	Indications	Dose regimens
Linezolid	Pneumonia Nosocomial pneumonia caused by *Staphylococcus aureus* (methicillin-susceptible and -resistant isolates) or Streptococcus pneumoniae. Community-acquired pneumonia caused by Streptococcus pneumoniae, including cases with concurrent bacteremia, or *Staphylococcus aureus* (methicillin-susceptible isolates only) Skin and Skin Structure Infections Complicated skin and skin structure infections, including diabetic foot infections, without concomitant osteomyelitis, caused by *Staphylococcus aureus* (methicillin-susceptible and -resistant isolates), Streptococcus pyogenes, or Streptococcus agalactiae. Linezolid has not been studied in the treatment of decubitus ulcers. Uncomplicated skin and skin structure infections caused by *Staphylococcus aureus* (methicillin-susceptible isolates only) or Streptococcus pyogenes. Vancomycin-Resistant Enterococcus Faecium Infections including cases with concurrent bacteremia.	Adults: 600 mg intravenously every 12 hours Pediatrics: 10 mg/kg intravenously every 8 or 12 h
Daptomycin	Complicated Skin And Skin Structure Infections Complicated skin and skin structure infections (cSSSI) caused by susceptible isolates of the following Gram-positive bacteria: *Staphylococcus aureus* (including methicillin-resistant isolates), Streptococcus pyogenes, Streptococcus agalactiae, Streptococcus dysgalactiae subsp. equisimilis, and	Adults: 4 mg/k (ABSSSI) or 6 mg/kg (bacteremia including right sided endocarditis) should be administered intravenously in 0.9% sodium chloride injection once every 24 hours Pediatrics:

Drug	Indications	Dose regimens
	Enterococcus faecalis (vancomycin-susceptible isolates only). *Staphylococcus aureus* Bloods tream Infections (Bacteremia), Including Those with Right-Sided Infective Endocarditis, Caused by Methicillin-Susceptible and Methicillin-Resistant Isolates.	Not approved
Ceftaroline	Acute Bacterial Skin And Skin Structure Infections Ceftaroline is indicated for the treatment of acute bacterial skin and skin structure infections (ABSSSI) caused by susceptible isolates of the following Gram-positive and Gram-negative microorganisms: *Staphylococcus aureus* (including methicillin-susceptible and -resistant isolates), Streptococcus pyogenes, Streptococcus agalactiae, Escherichia coli, Klebsiella pneumoniae, and Klebsiella oxytoca. Community-Acquired Bacterial Pneumonia Ceftaroline is indicated for the treatment of community-acquired bacterial pneumonia (CABP) caused by susceptible isolates of the following Gram-positive and Gram-negative microorganisms: Streptococcus pneumoniae (including cases with concurrent bacteremia), *Staphylococcus aureus* (methicillin-susceptible isolates only), Haemophilus influenzae, Klebsiella pneumoniae, Klebsiella oxytoca, and Escherichia coli.	Adults: 600 mg ever 12 h infusion over 5 to 60 minutes Pediatrics: Pediatric patients from 2 years to < 18 years of age weighing ≤ 33 kg: 12 mg/kg every 8 hours by IV infusion administered over 5 to 60 min. Pediatric patients from 2 years to < 18 years of age weighing > 33 kg: 400 mg every 8 hours or 600 mg every 12 hours by IV infusion administered over 5 to 60 min Pediatric patients from 2 months to < 2 years of age: 8 mg/kg every 8 hours by IV infusion administered over 5 to 60 min

REFERENCES

American Thoracic, Society, and America Infectious Diseases Society of. 2005. "Guidelines for the management of adults with hospital-acquired, ventilator-associated, and healthcare-associated pneumonia." *Am J Respir Crit Care Med* 171 (4): 388-416. https://doi.org/10.1164/rccm.200405-644ST. https://www.ncbi.nlm.nih.gov/pubmed/1569909 79.

Anderson, D. J., and K. S. Kaye. 2009. "Staphylococcal surgical site infections." *Infect Dis Clin North Am* 23 (1): 53-72. https://doi.org/10.1016/j.idc.2008.10.004. https://www.ncbi.nlm.nih.gov/pubmed/19135916.

Antonov, N. K., M. C. Garzon, K. D. Morel, S. Whittier, P. J. Planet, and C. T. Lauren. 2015. "High prevalence of mupirocin resistance in *Staphylococcus aureus* isolates from a pediatric population." *Antimicrob Agents Chemother* 59 (6): 3350-6. https://doi.org/10.1128/AAC.00079-15. https://www.ncbi.nlm.nih.gov/pubmed/25824213.

Bamberger, D. M. 2007. "Bacteremia and endocarditis due to methicillin-resistant *Staphylococcus aureus*: the potential role of daptomycin." *Ther Clin Risk Manag* 3 (4): 675-84. https://www.ncbi.nlm.nih.gov/pubmed/18472990.

Bamgbola, O. 2016. "Review of vancomycin-induced renal toxicity: an update." *Ther Adv Endocrinol Metab* 7 (3): 136-47. https://doi.org/10.1177/2042018816638223. https://www.ncbi.nlm.nih.gov/pubmed/27293542.

Bangert, S., M. Levy, and A. A. Hebert. 2012. "Bacterial resistance and impetigo treatment trends: a review." *Pediatr Dermatol* 29 (3): 243-8. https://doi.org/10.1111/j.1525-1470.2011.01700.x. https://www.ncbi.nlm.nih.gov/pubmed/22299710.

Bassetti, M., M. Peghin, E. M. Trecarichi, A. Carnelutti, E. Righi, P. Del Giacomo, F. Ansaldi, C. Trucchi, C. Alicino, R. Cauda, A. Sartor, T. Spanu, C. Scarparo, and M. Tumbarello. 2017. "Characteristics of *Staphylococcus aureus* Bacteraemia and Predictors of Early and Late Mortality." *PLoS One* 12 (2): e0170236. https://doi.org/10.1371/

journal.pone.0170236. https://www.ncbi.nlm.nih.gov/pubmed/28152067.

Bowen, A. C., J. R. Carapetis, B. J. Currie, V. Fowler, Jr., H. F. Chambers, and S. Y. C. Tong. 2017. "Sulfamethoxazole-Trimethoprim (Cotrimoxazole) for Skin and Soft Tissue Infections Including Impetigo, Cellulitis, and Abscess." *Open Forum Infect Dis* 4 (4): ofx232. https://doi.org/10.1093/ofid/ofx232. https://www.ncbi.nlm.nih.gov/pubmed/29255730.

Brown, E. M., and P. Thomas. 2002. "Fusidic acid resistance in *Staphylococcus aureus* isolates." *Lancet* 359 (9308): 803. https://doi.org/10.1016/S0140-6736(02)07869-8. https://www.ncbi.nlm.nih.gov/pubmed/11888633.

Brown, Justin, David L. Shriner, Robert A. Schwartz, and Camila K. Janniger. 2003. "Impetigo: an update." *International journal of dermatology* 42 (4): 251-255. https://doi.org/10.1046/j.1365-4362.2003.01647.x. https://pubmed.ncbi.nlm.nih.gov/12694487.

Cunha, B. A., N. Mikail, and L. Eisenstein. 2008. "Persistent methicillin-resistant *Staphylococcus aureus* (MRSA) bacteremia due to a linezolid "tolerant" strain." *Heart Lung* 37 (5): 398-400. https://doi.org/10.1016/j.hrtlng.2007.12.001. https://www.ncbi.nlm.nih.gov/pubmed/18790342.

Dagan, R., and Y. Bar-David. 1992. "Double-blind study comparing erythromycin and mupirocin for treatment of impetigo in children: implications of a high prevalence of erythromycin-resistant *Staphylococcus aureus* strains." *Antimicrob Agents Chemother* 36 (2): 287-90. https://doi.org/10.1128/aac.36.2.287. https://www.ncbi.nlm.nih.gov/pubmed/1605593.

Darmstadt, G. L., and A. T. Lane. 1994. "Impetigo: an overview." *Pediatr Dermatol* 11 (4): 293-303. https://doi.org/10.1111/j.1525-1470.1994.tb00092.x. https://www.ncbi.nlm.nih.gov/pubmed/7899177.

Dehority, W., E. Wang, P. S. Vernon, C. Lee, F. Perdreau-Remington, and J. Bradley. 2006. "Community-associated methicillin-resistant *Staphylococcus aureus* necrotizing fasciitis in a neonate." *Pediatr Infect*

Dis J 25 (11): 1080-1. https://doi.org/10.1097/01.inf.0000243158.25713.29. https://www.ncbi.nlm.nih.gov/pubmed/17072137.

DeSena, H. C., R. W. Steele, and T. W. Young. 2010. "Shock and persistent MRSA bacteremia." *Clin Pediatr (Phila)* 49 (5): 509-11. https://doi.org/10.1177/0009922809351741. https://www.ncbi.nlm.nih.gov/pubmed/20118078.

Dobie, D., and J. Gray. 2004. "Fusidic acid resistance in *Staphylococcus aureus*." *Arch Dis Child* 89 (1): 74-7. https://doi.org/10.1136/adc.2003.019695. https://www.ncbi.nlm.nih.gov/pubmed/14709515.

Eckmann, C., and M. Dryden. 2010. "Treatment of complicated skin and soft-tissue infections caused by resistant bacteria: value of linezolid, tigecycline, daptomycin and vancomycin." *Eur J Med Res* 15 (12): 554-63. https://doi.org/10.1186/2047-783x-15-12-554. https://www.ncbi.nlm.nih.gov/pubmed/21163730.

Eriksen, K. R. 1961. "["Celbenin"-resistant staphylococci]." *Ugeskr Laeger* 123: 384-6. https://www.ncbi.nlm.nih.gov/pubmed/13697147.

Fernandes, P. 2016. "Fusidic Acid: A Bacterial Elongation Factor Inhibitor for the Oral Treatment of Acute and Chronic Staphylococcal Infections." *Cold Spring Harb Perspect Med* 6 (1): a025437. https://doi.org/10.1101/cshperspect.a025437. https://www.ncbi.nlm.nih.gov/pubmed/26729758.

Fitch, M. T., D. E. Manthey, H. D. McGinnis, B. A. Nicks, and M. Pariyadath. 2007. "Videos in clinical medicine. Abscess incision and drainage." *N Engl J Med* 357 (19): e20. https://doi.org/10.1056/NEJMvcm071319. https://www.ncbi.nlm.nih.gov/pubmed/17989377.

Forestier, E., V. Remy, M. Mohseni-Zadeh, O. Lesens, B. Jauhlac, D. Christmann, and Y. Hansmann. 2007. "[MRSA bacteremia: recent epidemiological and therapeutical trends]." *Rev Med Interne* 28 (11): 746-55. https://doi.org/10.1016/j.revmed.2006.11.014. https://www.ncbi.nlm.nih.gov/pubmed/17513023.

Frank R. DeLeo, Binh An Diep, Michael Otto. 2009. "Host Defense and Pathogenesis in *Staphylococcus aureus* Infections." *Infectious Disease Clinics of North America* 23 (1): 17-34.

Geria, Aanand N., and Robert A. Schwartz. 2010. "Impetigo update: new challenges in the era of methicillin resistance." *Cutis* 85 (2): 65-70. https://pubmed.ncbi.nlm.nih.gov/20349679.

Hartman-Adams, H., C. Banvard, and G. Juckett. 2014. "Impetigo: diagnosis and treatment." *Am Fam Physician* 90 (4): 229-35. https://www.ncbi.nlm.nih.gov/pubmed/25250996.

Hassoun, A., P. K. Linden, and B. Friedman. 2017. "Incidence, prevalence, and management of MRSA bacteremia across patient populations-a review of recent developments in MRSA management and treatment." *Crit Care* 21 (1): 211. https://doi.org/10.1186/s13054-017-1801-3. https://www.ncbi.nlm.nih.gov/pubmed/28807042.

Jacobs, M. R., and P. C. Appelbaum. 2006. "Nadifloxacin: a quinolone for topical treatment of skin infections and potential for systemic use of its active isomer, WCK 771." *Expert Opin Pharmacother* 7 (14): 1957-66. https://doi.org/10.1517/14656566.7.14.1957. https://www.ncbi.nlm.nih.gov/pubmed/17020421.

Jayaweera, A. S., M. Karunarathne, W. W. Kumbukgolla, and H. L. Thushari. 2017. "Prevalence of methicillin resistant *Staphylococcus aureus* (MRSA) bacteremia at Teaching Hospital Anuradhapura, Sri Lanka." *Ceylon Med J* 62 (2): 110-111. https://doi.org/10.4038/cmj.v62i2.8478. https://www.ncbi.nlm.nih.gov/pubmed/28699335.

Kavanagh, N., E. J. Ryan, A. Widaa, G. Sexton, J. Fennell, S. O'Rourke, K. C. Cahill, C. J. Kearney, F. J. O'Brien, and S. W. Kerrigan. 2018. "Staphylococcal Osteomyelitis: Disease Progression, Treatment Challenges, and Future Directions." *Clin Microbiol Rev* 31 (2). https://doi.org/10.1128/CMR.00084-17. https://www.ncbi.nlm.nih.gov/pubmed/29444953.

Kempker, R. R., M. M. Farley, J. L. Ladson, S. Satola, and S. M. Ray. 2010. "Association of methicillin-resistant *Staphylococcus aureus* (MRSA) USA300 genotype with mortality in MRSA bacteremia." *J Infect* 61 (5): 372-81. https://doi.org/10.1016/j.jinf.2010.09.021. https://www.ncbi.nlm.nih.gov/pubmed/20868707.

Khawcharoenporn, T., and A. Tice. 2010. "Empiric outpatient therapy with trimethoprim-sulfamethoxazole, cephalexin, or clindamycin for cellulitis." *Am J Med* 123 (10): 942-50. https://doi.org/10.1016/j.amjmed.2010.05.020. https://www.ncbi.nlm.nih.gov/pubmed/20920697.

Kobayashi, S. D., N. Malachowa, and F. R. DeLeo. 2015. "Pathogenesis of *Staphylococcus aureus* abscesses." *Am J Pathol* 185 (6): 1518-27. https://doi.org/10.1016/j.ajpath.2014.11.030. https://www.ncbi.nlm.nih.gov/pubmed/25749135.

Koning, S., J. C. van der Wouden, O. Chosidow, M. Twynholm, K. P. Singh, N. Scangarella, and A. P. Oranje. 2008. "Efficacy and safety of retapamulin ointment as treatment of impetigo: randomized double-blind multicentre placebo-controlled trial." *Br J Dermatol* 158 (5): 1077-82. https://doi.org/10.1111/j.1365-2133.2008.08485.x. https://www.ncbi.nlm.nih.gov/pubmed/18341664.

Koning, S., L. W. van Suijlekom-Smit, J. L. Nouwen, C. M. Verduin, R. M. Bernsen, A. P. Oranje, S. Thomas, and J. C. van der Wouden. 2002. "Fusidic acid cream in the treatment of impetigo in general practice: double blind randomised placebo controlled trial." *BMJ* 324 (7331): 203-6. https://doi.org/10.1136/bmj.324.7331.203. https://www.ncbi.nlm.nih.gov/pubmed/11809642.

Lacey, Keenan A., Joan A. Geoghegan, and Rachel M. McLoughlin. 2016. "The Role of *Staphylococcus aureus* Virulence Factors in Skin Infection and Their Potential as Vaccine Antigens." *Pathogens (Basel, Switzerland)* 5 (1): 22. https://doi.org/10.3390/pathogens5010022. https://pubmed.ncbi.nlm.nih.gov/26901227; https://www.ncbi.nlm.nih.gov/pmc/articles/PMC4810143/.

Lee, C. C., P. L. Chen, L. R. Wang, H. C. Lee, C. M. Chang, N. Y. Lee, C. J. Wu, H. I. Shih, and W. C. Ko. 2006. "Fatal case of community-acquired bacteremia and necrotizing fasciitis caused by *Chryseobacterium meningosepticum*: case report and review of the literature." *J Clin Microbiol* 44 (3): 1181-3. https://doi.org/10.1128/JCM.44.3.1181-1183.2006. https://www.ncbi.nlm.nih.gov/pubmed/16517926.

Lee, C. Y., H. C. Tsai, C. M. Kunin, S. S. Lee, and Y. S. Chen. 2015. "Clinical and microbiological characteristics of purulent and non-purulent cellulitis in hospitalized Taiwanese adults in the era of community-associated methicillin-resistant *Staphylococcus aureus*." *BMC Infect Dis* 15: 311. https://doi.org/10.1186/s12879-015-1064-z. https://www.ncbi.nlm.nih.gov/pubmed/26242240.

Lee, Y. T., J. C. Lin, N. C. Wang, M. Y. Peng, and F. Y. Chang. 2007. "Necrotizing fasciitis in a medical center in northern Taiwan: emergence of methicillin-resistant *Staphylococcus aureus* in the community." *J Microbiol Immunol Infect* 40 (4): 335-41. https://www.ncbi.nlm.nih.gov/pubmed/17712468.

Levin, T. P., B. Suh, P. Axelrod, A. L. Truant, and T. Fekete. 2005. "Potential clindamycin resistance in clindamycin-susceptible, erythromycin-resistant *Staphylococcus aureus*: report of a clinical failure." *Antimicrob Agents Chemother* 49 (3): 1222-4. https://doi.org/10.1128/AAC.49.3.1222-1224.2005. https://www.ncbi.nlm.nih.gov/pubmed/15728934.

Liu, C., A. Bayer, S. E. Cosgrove, R. S. Daum, S. K. Fridkin, R. J. Gorwitz, S. L. Kaplan, A. W. Karchmer, D. P. Levine, B. E. Murray, J. Rybak M, D. A. Talan, and H. F. Chambers. 2011. "Clinical practice guidelines by the infectious diseases society of America for the treatment of methicillin-resistant *Staphylococcus aureus* infections in adults and children: executive summary." *Clin Infect Dis* 52 (3): 285-92. https://doi.org/10.1093/cid/cir034. https://www.ncbi.nlm.nih.gov/pubmed/21217178.

Moellering, R. C., Jr. 2012. "MRSA: the first half century." *J Antimicrob Chemother* 67 (1): 4-11. https://doi.org/10.1093/jac/dkr437. https://www.ncbi.nlm.nih.gov/pubmed/22010206.

Moise, P. A., D. L. Culshaw, A. Wong-Beringer, J. Bensman, K. C. Lamp, W. J. Smith, K. Bauer, D. A. Goff, R. Adamson, K. Leuthner, M. D. Virata, J. A. McKinnell, S. B. Chaudhry, R. Eskandarian, T. Lodise, K. Reyes, and M. J. Zervos. 2016. "Comparative Effectiveness of Vancomycin Versus Daptomycin for MRSA Bacteremia With Vancomycin MIC >1 mg/L: A Multicenter Evaluation." *Clin Ther* 38

(1): 16-30. https://doi.org/10.1016/j.clinthera.2015.09.017. https://www.ncbi.nlm.nih.gov/pubmed/26585355.

Mruk, A. L., and K. E. Record. 2012. "Antimicrobial options in the treatment of adult staphylococcal bone and joint infections in an era of drug shortages." *Orthopedics* 35 (5): 401-7. https://doi.org/10.3928/01477447-20120426-07. https://www.ncbi.nlm.nih.gov/pubmed/22588396.

Nair, S. P., R. J. Williams, and B. Henderson. 2000. "Advances in our understanding of the bone and joint pathology caused by *Staphylococcus aureus* infection." *Rheumatology (Oxford)* 39 (8): 821-34. https://doi.org/10.1093/rheumatology/39.8.821. https://www.ncbi.nlm.nih.gov/pubmed/10952735.

Narayanan, V., S. Motlekar, G. Kadhe, and S. Bhagat. 2014. "Efficacy and safety of nadifloxacin for bacterial skin infections: results from clinical and post-marketing studies." *Dermatol Ther (Heidelb)* 4 (2): 233-48. https://doi.org/10.1007/s13555-014-0062-1. https://www.ncbi.nlm.nih.gov/pubmed/25212256.

Nenoff, P., U. F. Haustein, and N. Hittel. 2004. "Activity of nadifloxacin (OPC-7251) and seven other antimicrobial agents against aerobic and anaerobic Gram-positive bacteria isolated from bacterial skin infections." *Chemotherapy* 50 (4): 196-201. https://doi.org/10.1159/000081032. https://www.ncbi.nlm.nih.gov/pubmed/15452398.

Nichols, R. L., and S. Florman. 2001. "Clinical presentations of soft-tissue infections and surgical site infections." *Clin Infect Dis* 33 Suppl 2: S84-93. https://doi.org/10.1086/321862. https://www.ncbi.nlm.nih.gov/pubmed/11486304.

Oranje, A. P., O. Chosidow, S. Sacchidanand, G. Todd, K. Singh, N. Scangarella, R. Shawar, M. Twynholm, and T. O. C. Study Team. 2007. "Topical retapamulin ointment, 1%, versus sodium fusidate ointment, 2%, for impetigo: a randomized, observer-blinded, noninferiority study." *Dermatology* 215 (4): 331-40. https://doi.org/10.1159/000107776. https://www.ncbi.nlm.nih.gov/pubmed/17911992.

Ortwine, J. K., and K. Bhavan. 2018. "Morbidity, mortality, and management of methicillin-resistant *S. aureus* bacteremia in the USA:

update on antibacterial choices and understanding." *Hosp Pract (1995)* 46 (2): 64-72. https://doi.org/10.1080/21548331.2018.1435128. https://www.ncbi.nlm.nih.gov/pubmed/29400119.

osé Romero-Vivas, Margarita Rubio, Cristina Fernandez, Juan J. Picazo. 1995. "Mortality Associated with Nosocomial Bacteremia Due to Methicillin-Resistant *Staphylococcus aureus.*" *Clinical Infectious Diseases* 21 (6): 1417–1423.

Owens, C. D., and K. Stoessel. 2008. "Surgical site infections: epidemiology, microbiology and prevention." *J Hosp Infect* 70 Suppl 2: 3-10. https://doi.org/10.1016/S0195-6701(08)60017-1. https://www.ncbi.nlm.nih.gov/pubmed/19022115.

Pastagia, M., L. C. Kleinman, E. G. Lacerda de la Cruz, and S. G. Jenkins. 2012. "Predicting risk for death from MRSA bacteremia." *Emerg Infect Dis* 18 (7): 1072-80. https://doi.org/10.3201/eid1807.101371. https://www.ncbi.nlm.nih.gov/pubmed/22709685.

Patel, J. B., R. J. Gorwitz, and J. A. Jernigan. 2009. "Mupirocin resistance." *Clin Infect Dis* 49 (6): 935-41. https://doi.org/10.1086/605495. https://www.ncbi.nlm.nih.gov/pubmed/19673644.

Peng, H., D. Liu, Y. Ma, and W. Gao. 2018. "Comparison of community- and healthcare-associated methicillin-resistant *Staphylococcus aureus* isolates at a Chinese tertiary hospital, 2012-2017." *Sci Rep* 8 (1): 17916. https://doi.org/10.1038/s41598-018-36206-5. https://www.ncbi.nlm.nih.gov/pubmed/30559468.

Poovelikunnel, T., G. Gethin, and H. Humphreys. 2015. "Mupirocin resistance: clinical implications and potential alternatives for the eradication of MRSA." *J Antimicrob Chemother* 70 (10): 2681-92. https://doi.org/10.1093/jac/dkv169. https://www.ncbi.nlm.nih.gov/pubmed/26142407.

Popovich, K. J., R. A. Weinstein, and B. Hota. 2008. "Are community-associated methicillin-resistant *Staphylococcus aureus* (MRSA) strains replacing traditional nosocomial MRSA strains?" *Clin Infect Dis* 46 (6): 787-94. https://doi.org/10.1086/528716. https://www.ncbi.nlm.nih.gov/pubmed/18266611.

Prabhoo, R., R. Chaddha, R. Iyer, A. Mehra, J. Ahdal, and R. Jain. 2019. "Overview of methicillin resistant *Staphylococcus aureus* mediated bone and joint infections in India." *Orthop Rev (Pavia)* 11 (2): 8070. https://doi.org/10.4081/or.2019.8070. https://www.ncbi.nlm.nih.gov/pubmed/31312419.

Raff, A. B., and D. Kroshinsky. 2016. "Cellulitis: A Review." *JAMA* 316 (3): 325-37. https://doi.org/10.1001/jama.2016.8825. https://www.ncbi.nlm.nih.gov/pubmed/27434444.

Rubinstein, E., M. H. Kollef, and D. Nathwani. 2008. "Pneumonia caused by methicillin-resistant *Staphylococcus aureus*." *Clin Infect Dis* 46 Suppl 5: S378-85. https://doi.org/10.1086/533594. https://www.ncbi.nlm.nih.gov/pubmed/18462093.

Rybak, M., B. Lomaestro, J. C. Rotschafer, R. Moellering, Jr., W. Craig, M. Billeter, J. R. Dalovisio, and D. P. Levine. 2009. "Therapeutic monitoring of vancomycin in adult patients: a consensus review of the American Society of Health-System Pharmacists, the Infectious Diseases Society of America, and the Society of Infectious Diseases Pharmacists." *Am J Health Syst Pharm* 66 (1): 82-98. https://doi.org/10.2146/ajhp080434. https://www.ncbi.nlm.nih.gov/pubmed/19106348.

Schofer, H., and L. Simonsen. 2010. "Fusidic acid in dermatology: an updated review." *Eur J Dermatol* 20 (1): 6-15. https://doi.org/10.1684/ejd.2010.0833. https://www.ncbi.nlm.nih.gov/pubmed/20007058.

Shallcross, Laura J., Ellen Fragaszy, Anne M. Johnson, and Andrew C. Hayward. 2013. "The role of the Panton-Valentine leucocidin toxin in staphylococcal disease: a systematic review and meta-analysis." *The Lancet. Infectious diseases* 13 (1): 43-54. https://doi.org/10.1016/S1473-3099(12)70238-4. https://pubmed.ncbi.nlm.nih.gov/23103172. https://www.ncbi.nlm.nih.gov/pmc/articles/PMC3530297/.

Sheftel, T. G., J. T. Mader, J. J. Pennick, and G. Cierny, 3rd. 1985. "Methicillin-resistant *Staphylococcus aureus* osteomyelitis." *Clin Orthop Relat Res* (198): 231-9. https://www.ncbi.nlm.nih.gov/pubmed/4028555.

Silverman, J. A., L. I. Mortin, A. D. Vanpraagh, T. Li, and J. Alder. 2005. "Inhibition of daptomycin by pulmonary surfactant: in vitro modeling and clinical impact." *J Infect Dis* 191 (12): 2149-52. https://doi.org/10.1086/430352. https://www.ncbi.nlm.nih.gov/pubmed/15898002.

Sit, P. S., C. S. J. Teh, N. Idris, and S. Ponnampalavanar. 2018. "Methicillin-resistant *Staphylococcus aureus* (MRSA) bacteremia: Correlations between clinical, phenotypic, genotypic characteristics and mortality in a tertiary teaching hospital in Malaysia." *Infect Genet Evol* 59: 132-141. https://doi.org/10.1016/j.meegid.2018.01.031. https://www.ncbi.nlm.nih.gov/pubmed/29421224.

Spellberg, B., and B. A. Lipsky. 2012. "Systemic antibiotic therapy for chronic osteomyelitis in adults." *Clin Infect Dis* 54 (3): 393-407. https://doi.org/10.1093/cid/cir842. https://www.ncbi.nlm.nih.gov/pubmed/22157324.

Tadros, M., V. Williams, B. L. Coleman, A. J. McGeer, S. Haider, C. Lee, H. Iacovides, E. Rubinstein, M. John, L. Johnston, S. McNeil, K. Katz, N. Laffin, K. N. Suh, J. Powis, S. Smith, G. Taylor, C. Watt, and A. E. Simor. 2013. "Epidemiology and outcome of pneumonia caused by methicillin-resistant *Staphylococcus aureus* (MRSA) in Canadian hospitals." *PLoS One* 8 (9): e75171. https://doi.org/10.1371/journal.pone.0075171. https://www.ncbi.nlm.nih.gov/pubmed/24069391.

Tong, S. Y., J. S. Davis, E. Eichenberger, T. L. Holland, and V. G. Fowler, Jr. 2015. "*Staphylococcus aureus* infections: epidemiology, pathophysiology, clinical manifestations, and management." *Clin Microbiol Rev* 28 (3): 603-61. https://doi.org/10.1128/CMR.00134-14. https://www.ncbi.nlm.nih.gov/pubmed/26016486.

Urushibara, N., M. S. Aung, M. Kawaguchiya, and N. Kobayashi. 2020. "Novel staphylococcal cassette chromosome mec (SCCmec) type XIV (5A) and a truncated SCCmec element in SCC composite islands carrying speG in ST5 MRSA in Japan." *J Antimicrob Chemother* 75 (1): 46-50. https://doi.org/10.1093/jac/dkz406. https://www.ncbi.nlm.nih.gov/pubmed/31617906.

Vera, R. Mario. 2017. "Management of Surgical Site Infections " In *Common Problems in Acute Care Surgery*. Switzerland: Springer International Publishing.

Weigelt, J. A., B. A. Lipsky, Y. P. Tabak, K. G. Derby, M. Kim, and V. Gupta. 2010. "Surgical site infections: Causative pathogens and associated outcomes." *Am J Infect Control* 38 (2): 112-20. https://doi.org/10.1016/j.ajic.2009.06.010. https://www.ncbi.nlm.nih.gov/pubmed/19889474.

Weigelt, J., H. M. Kaafarani, K. M. Itani, and R. N. Swanson. 2004. "Linezolid eradicates MRSA better than vancomycin from surgical-site infections." *Am J Surg* 188 (6): 760-6. https://doi.org/10.1016/j.amjsurg.2004.08.045. https://www.ncbi.nlm.nih.gov/pubmed/15619496.

Wilkinson, J. D. 1998. "Fusidic acid in dermatology." *Br J Dermatol* 139 Suppl 53: 37-40. https://doi.org/10.1046/j.1365-2133.1998.1390s3037.x. https://www.ncbi.nlm.nih.gov/pubmed/9990411.

Woodford, N., M. Afzal-Shah, M. Warner, and D. M. Livermore. 2008. "In vitro activity of retapamulin against *Staphylococcus aureus* isolates resistant to fusidic acid and mupirocin." *J Antimicrob Chemother* 62 (4): 766-8. https://doi.org/10.1093/jac/dkn266. https://www.ncbi.nlm.nih.gov/pubmed/18567573.

Yang, C. C., C. L. Sy, Y. C. Huang, S. S. Shie, J. C. Shu, P. H. Hsieh, C. H. Hsiao, and C. J. Chen. 2018. "Risk factors of treatment failure and 30-day mortality in patients with bacteremia due to MRSA with reduced vancomycin susceptibility." *Sci Rep* 8 (1): 7868. https://doi.org/10.1038/s41598-018-26277-9. https://www.ncbi.nlm.nih.gov/pubmed/29777150.

Ye, Z. K., Y. L. Chen, K. Chen, X. L. Zhang, G. H. Du, B. He, D. K. Li, Y. N. Liu, K. H. Yang, Y. Y. Zhang, S. D. Zhai, the Guideline Development Group Guideline Steering Group, and Group the Guideline Secretary. 2016. "Therapeutic drug monitoring of vancomycin: a guideline of the Division of Therapeutic Drug Monitoring, Chinese Pharmacological Society." *J Antimicrob Chemother* 71 (11): 3020-3025.

https://doi.org/10.1093/jac/dkw254. https://www.ncbi.nlm.nih.gov/pubmed/27494905.

Ye, Z. K., C. Li, and S. D. Zhai. 2014. "Guidelines for therapeutic drug monitoring of vancomycin: a systematic review." *PLoS One* 9 (6): e99044. https://doi.org/10.1371/journal.pone.0099044. https://www.ncbi.nlm.nih.gov/pubmed/24932495.

In: Methicillin-Resistant Staphylococcus ... ISBN: 978-1-53618-189-0
Editor: Erick Pereira Alves © 2020 Nova Science Publishers, Inc.

Chapter 4

AN OVERVIEW ON PATHOGENESIS AND TREATMENT OF METHICILLIN-RESISTANT *STAPHYLOCOCCUS AUREUS* (MRSA)

*Ritika Chauhan and Jayanthi Abraham**
Microbial Biotechnology Laboratory,
School of Biosciences and Technology,
VIT University, Vellore, Tamil Nadu

ABSTRACT

Staphylococcus is a natural inhabitant of the skin and nasal cavities of almost 30 percent of the healthy population. The *Staphylococcus* strains which have developed resistance towards penicillin-related drugs such as amoxicillin and methicillin are known as methicillin-resistant *Staphylococcus aureus* (MRSA). The emergence and various outbreaks of MRSA over the decades have made it difficult to combat antibiotic resistance with the current class of antibiotics. The major causes for prevalence of MRSA are the increasing hospital-associated bacterial infections (HA-MRSA), health care associated MRSA-patients with

---

* Corresponding Author's E-mail: jayanthi.abraham@gmail.com.

ongoing dialysis or chemotherapy and also community associated MRSA-transfer from human to human transmission. The present book chapter emphasizes the occurrence of MRSA in health care settings as well as community-based infections, the symptoms and diagnosis associated with MRSA infections, treatment and various mechanisms to combat methicillin resistant *Staphylococcus aureus*.

Keywords: MRSA, antibiotic resistance, penicillin, nosocomial infections

INTRODUCTION

Staphylococcus aureus is a Gram-positive coccus, organised in grape-like clusters. It is part of the natural microbiota of the human body, residing mainly on the skin, armpit, nasal cavity, and upper respiratory tract. Being a natural habitat of the human body, most of the time *Staphylococcus aureus* acts as a commensal of human microbiota and is harmless. However, they are opportunistic pathogens and infections caused by them can be fatal (Lowry, 1998). The infections caused by *Staphylococcus aureus* is of public health concern because almost 20-40% of the healthy population are carriers, which increases the epidemiological risk from various continents across the globe (Kozada et al., 2019). As an opportunistic pathogen, *Staphylococcus aureus* infections caused by soft tissue injuries, open wounds, bacteremia or sepsis, pneumonia, endocarditis, and osteomyelitis can be lethal. People of any age group can develop infections but certain groups of people are at higher risk, such as patients with infections or chronic conditions and hospital staff.

Hospital staff and patients who: are in intensive care units (ICU), with catheters, have prosthetic devices, various infections, or chronic conditions, and drug users have increased risk (Taylor and Unakal 2019).

Staphylococcus aureus strains which have developed resistance to Beta-lactam antibiotics-penicillin, cephalosporins, and carbapenems are known as Methicillin-resistant *Staphylococcus aureus* (MRSA). With the introduction of penicillin in 1942, various staphylococcal infections became treatable. Unfortunately, resistance to the drug developed shortly after. Methicillin was developed in 1959 to act against staphylococcal strains resistant to penicillin. However, in 1961 *Staphylococcus aureus* acquired resistance against methicillin which was widespread in hospitals, and MRSA strains were confirmed from the United Kingdom, Japan, Australia and the United states. A pandemic was observed in 1970 and 1980 due to sudden increase in hospital acquired MRSA infections, which continues to impact morbidity and mortality in hospitals across the world (Chambers and DeLeo, 2009). The exceptional outbreak of MRSA infections transmitted between hospitals increased by 22% in 1995 and 50% in 1997 (Murray and Patrick 2007). According to the Centre of Disease Control (CDC), an estimate of 1,25,969 *Staphylococcus aureus* infected patients were admitted in hospitals during 1999-2000. It was found that 43% of *Staphylococcus aureus* isolates were methicillin resistant (Kuehnert et al., 2005). In 2003, almost 4,00,000 US citizens were admitted in hospitals due to MRSA infections (Noskin et al., 2007). In 2004, the National Nosocomial Infections Surveillance System (NNISS) reported that the number of health care-associated staphylococcal infections increased by 3.1% each year in ICUs due to MRSA. The increasing MRSA infections impose significant impact and burden on health care resources (Boucher and Corey 2008).

The infrequent HA-MRSA outbreaks created a lot of panic among health care workers due to its notable morbidity and mortality. The CA-MRSA was earlier predicted to be associated only with health care workers or people with prior healthcare exposure. Later, in 1993 MRSA isolates were found to be infective among Australian aborigines population who had no contact with the health care system (Udo et al., 1993). In 1997-1999, fatal MRSA infection was reported in four children by CDC in the United States (CDC 1999). In 2003, the Canadian MRSA surveillance system reported 5-7% of MRSA infections occurred in individuals with no health care background. CA-MRSA outbreaks were reported in athletes, children, prisoners, military personnel and new born infants by CDC in 1998-2005 (CDC 1999; 2003). The strains isolated from these patients were identified as community-associated strains both genotypically and phenotypically (Herold et al., 1998; Kallen et al., 2000; Eckhardt et al., 2003; Kazakova et al., 2005). It was clearly understood that infective staphylococcal strains in a community are not similar to hospital-associated staphylococcal strains, demonstrating the emergence of a unique community-associated staphylococcal infection. The prevalence of CA-MRSA is largely due to contact with uncovered wounds of individuals in crowded places, sharing personal hygiene items, drug usage, poor hygiene, and close skin-skin contact. Presently, MRSA is the leading cause of community associated staphylococcal infections.

Pathogenesis of MRSA

The colonization of *Staphylococcus aureus* in the anterior nares, (20-30% healthy population) nose, and throat are the major locations contributing to primary colonization. *Staphylococcus aureus* multiplies and colonizes these sites of healthy individuals, providing a reservoir from which bacteria can escape when an individual acquires a cut, abrasion, surgery, or any device insertion. Therefore, colonization is the risk factor for subsequent infection, and can be easily transmitted in healthcare as well as community settings. Although, the colonization of *S. aureus* is the underlying cause of various infections, *S. aureus* colonization is complex and not completely understood (Kluytmans et al., 1997; Wertheim et al., 2005; Gordon and Lowry 2008).

The surface proteins called "microbial surface components recognizing adhesive matrix molecules" (MSCRAMMs) of *Staphylococcus aureus* initiate the adherence to the host by binding host-tissue components and molecules including collagen, fibronectin, and fibrogen (Patti et al., 1994; Foster and Hook 1998). Once, *S. aureus* adheres to the host cell, it multiplies and continues to survive in the host. MSCRAMM plays a vital role in initiating staphylococcal infections such as endocarditis, septic arthritis, bone and joint infections, prosthetic-device infections, and catheter infections. The pathogenic strains of *S. aureus* rapidly produce biofilm on the host and on the surface of prosthetic devices which are introduced into the patients during or post-surgery. The biofilm formation by *S. aureus* on devices is difficult to treat or eradicate unless the device is replaced or removed from the patient (Tung et al., 2000; Donlan and Costerton 2002).

The intracellular persistence and recurrent *S. aureus* infections in the host are caused by small colony variants (SCVs) of *Staphylococcus aureus*. These bacterial variants are not particularly virulent but hide and survive as they bypass the antibiotic effect without causing any host cell damage. The patients suffering from cystic fibrosis (CF) and osteomyelitis are at higher risk of recurrent *S. aureus* SCVs infection because they suffer from chronic staphylococcal infection and long-term antibiotic therapy (Melter and Radojevic 2010).

Staphylococcus aureus is an opportunistic pathogen and elicits an inclusive set of virulence factors such as toxins, enzymes, adhesins and surface proteins that enhances the pathogen's ability to survive under unfavourable conditions, and remain persistent for a long period of time. The toxins or proteins secreted by *Staphylococcus aureus* penetrate the tissue and enables the bacteria to invade the host. Hemolysin, leukotoxin, exfoliative toxins, enterotoxin, and toxic shock syndrome toxin 1 are the most common toxins secreted by *S. aureus* (Kong et al., 2016). The hemolysin toxin lyses red blood cells and are categorized into α, β and γ-hemolysin. α-hemolysin is pore forming cytotoxin and performs its function by binding to its proteinaceous receptor ADAM10 and lyses rabbit red blood cells, but it is less effective against sheep and human erythrocytes (Wilke and Wardenburg 20110). β-hemolysin is a sphingomyelinase and non-pore forming toxin which hydrolyses sphingomyelin, and lyses monocytes and erythrocytes only at low temperature (Walev et al., 1996). γ-hemolysin is hemolytic to rabbit erythrocytes and also effective against leukocytes including neutrophils, monocytes, macrophages, and granulocytes (Vandenesch et al., 2012). The leukotoxins belong to the Luk-toxin family and the Panton-Valentine leukocidin (PVL) has been reported to be associated with CA-MRSA outbreaks (Otto 2010). The *Staphylococcus* enterotoxin (SE) is responsible for staphylococcal food poisoning which causes food-borne diseases characterised by nausea, vomiting, and diarrhoea after consumption of contaminated food. The toxins are secreted by entero-toxigenic *S. aureus* in food products, milk and milk products, and animal food such as meat and fish which are the major carriers of enterotoxins because this toxin is stable, even at 100°C. Cooked food left at room temperature gives an opportunity for *Staphylococcus* to colonize. *Staphylococcus* toxins are also called as super antigens which trigger T-cell activation and release of cytokines resulting in cell death via apoptosis or lethal toxic shock syndrome (TSS). The toxic shock syndrome toxins are lethal and lead to serious morbidity and mortality, also reported in women with regular use of tampons (Berkley et al., 1997). *Staphylococca*l exfoliative toxins (ETs) are the causative agent for staphylococcal scalded skin syndrome (SSSS), which appears as red blisters, burns or scald, or loss of superficial skin, commonly found in infants and neonates. The disrupted skin layer further facilitates colonization of bacteria and infection (Hanakawa et al., 2002). The major staphylococcus toxins-virulence factors are listed in Table 1.

Table 1. The function of *staphylococcus* virulence factors

Sl. No.	Toxin	Function
1	α-hemolysin	Cytotoxin, pore forming toxin, lysis the cell membrane, neurotoxin, toxic to macrophages, lysosomes, muscle tissue, renal cortex, circulatory system, lyses rabbit erythrocytes
2	β-hemolysin	Hemolytic for sheep cells, hydrolyses sphingomyelin
3	γ-hemolysin	Hemolytic to rabbit erythrocytes, damaging activity towards leucocytes
4	δ-hemolysin	Effects cell membrane of erythrocytes, leucocytes, macrophages and platelets, permeabilizes hydrophobic ceramide domains
5	Leukocidins	Bicomponent membrane-active toxins, PVL, damaging effects on leucocytes
6	Superantigens	Toxic shock syndrome associated with food borne diseases, tampon use, multiple organ failure and gastroenteritis
7	Exfoliative	Staphylococcal scalded skin syndrome associated with infants

HA-MRSA

The antimicrobial resistance in MRSA is mediated by horizontal gene transfer through certain elements such as plasmids, transposable genetic elements, and genomic islands (Jenson and Lyon 2009). The ability of MRSA to thrive in the presence of β-lactam antibiotics is due to the resistance gene *mecA*, which does not allow β-lactam antibiotics or enables cell-wall synthesis. Methicillin resistance is conferred by *mecA* gene, which encodes a penicillin-binding protein (PBP2A) that has low affinity for β-lactam antibiotics such as penicillins, cephalosporins, and carbapenems. Staphylococcal cassette chromosome *mec* (SCC*mec*) is a mobile genetic element and recombination site of staphylococcal species which harbours the *mecA* gene. This gene grants resistance to methicillin and channelizes antibiotic resistance through gene transfer. It has been proposed that SCCmec originated from a closely related species of *Staphylococcus sciuri*, and horizontally transferred to *Staphylococcus aureus* (Wu and Lencastre 2001). In addition, SCC*mec* contains other recombinase genes, like the cytolysin gene *psm-mec* (suppress virulence of HA-MRSA) *psm-mec*RNA, *ccrA/ccrB* or *ccC*, which permits intra-interspecies horizontal gene transfer (Kaito et al., 2011; Cheung et al., 2014).

The horizontal gene transfer through SCC*mec* in MRSA clones is the major cause for spread of HA-MRSA infections. The successful transfer of SCC*mec* into methicillin-susceptible staphylococcus strain (MSSA) gave rise to MRSA lineages with variable virulence (Gordon and Lowry 2008). Originally the MRSA clones emerged from five different groups of related genotypes. The first isolate evolved from sequence type (ST) 8-MSSA, which mutated and evolved into ST250-MSSA (first recipient of SCC*mec*) to yield ST250-MRSA-1 (first MRSA clone). Gordon and Lowry (2008) demonstrated the major MRSA clones responsible for spread of hospital-associated MRSA infections:

- ST2470-MRSA-1 (UK EMRSA-2, Iberian)
- ST239-MRSAIII (UK Epidemic MRSA-1)

- ST5-MRSAII (USA100, Glycopeptide Intermediate *Staphylococcus aureus*, Japanese)
- ST5-MRSAIV (USA800 and Paediatric)
- ST239-MRSA-III (UK-EMRSA-I, 4, 11, Brazilian, Portugese)
- ST8-MRSA-IV (USA300, USA500, UK Epidemic MRSA-2)
- ST45-MRSA-IV (Berlin and USA600)

These MRSA clones were disseminated across the globe and turned out to be the major cause of HA-MRSA infections. The emergence of strains EMRSA 15 and 16 causing nosocomial bacteremia in regions of the United Kingdom and Asia claimed many lives. In 1990, the virulent Brazilian clone also known as Brazilian epidemic clonal complex (BECC) was the major cause of staphylococcal infections in Joao Barros Barreto University Hospital, Brazil. This particular strain accounted for 79% of staphylococcal isolates by 1999 because of its ability for efficient adhesion, persistence and invasion of devices or epithelial cells to form biofilm (Amaral et al., 2005). With the spread of virulent strains MRSA clones were able to establish infections in hospital settings, but the spread of HA-MRSA infections across International borders which remain unclear. The disseminated strains must have established infection because of their ability to colonize hosts for a long time, enhanced virulence and increased transmissibility. The transmission of MRSA strains/MRSA clones among community and hospital settings is depicted in Figure 1.

The increasing spread of HA-MRSA can be prevented by control strategies such as active MRSA surveillance testing. When MRSA transmission rates are not decreasing, hand-hygiene, through environmental and equipment cleaning and decontamination are to be practised. Educating health workers, patients, and their family members, are the major decolonization strategies for MRSA and maintaining contact precautions. Figure 2 represents the control measures to prevent the spread of MRSA clones from hospital to community settings.

An Overview on Pathogenesis and Treatment ...   163

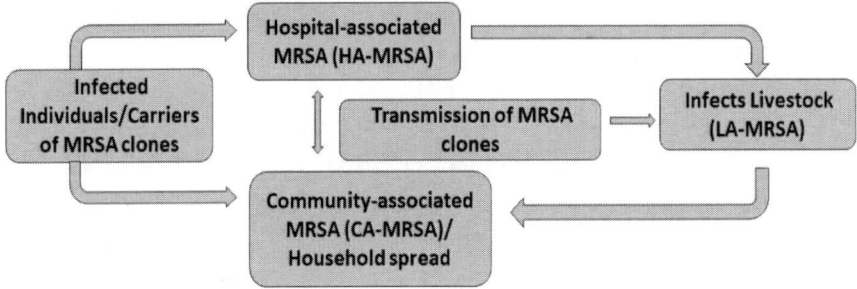

Figure 1. Transmission and spread of MRSA clones among community and hospital settings.

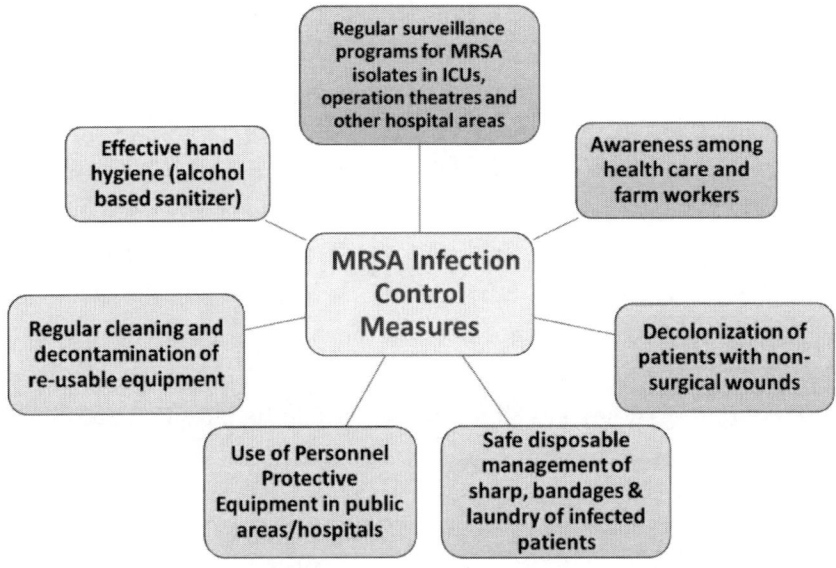

Figure 2. Preventive measures to control the spread of MRSA infections in community settings.

CA-MRSA

The CA-MRSA strains emerged in late 1990 infecting the set of people who were never exposed to health care settings, which indicates that CA-MRSA has not evolved from HA-MRSA. This was further confirmed by molecular-typing studies (Daum 2007). The CA-MRSA strains carry

SCC*mec*IV, the smallest of SCCs that confers methicillin resistance, but are susceptible to non-β-lactam antibiotics. On the other hand, HA-MRSA carries larger SCCmec types confirming the emergence of CA-MRSA not related with HA-MRSA strains (Zetolo et al., 2005; Ito et al., 2004). There were several outbreaks of CA-MRSA in 1990-2000 due to ST1 infections (also known as MW2 strain or USA400). Most of the fatal cases were ~~fatal~~ associated with necrotizing pneumonia or abscesses and sepsis. The strain was found to not only be infectious in humans, but also in animals due to its higher virulence. The virulence associated with MW2/USA400 strain was identified by comparing its sequence with the other virulent strains including N315-Japanese MRSA, Mu50-Vancomycin resistance MRSA, EMRSA-Epidemic resistance MRSA in UK, and NCTC8325. The presence of the Panton-Valentine Leukocidin (PVL) gene was the unique feature of this strain. The PVL gene in staphylococcus isolates represents increased virulence and is commonly found in CA-MRSA infections. Except PVL genes, MW2 strains were reported to possess 16 unique superantigen genes, 11 exotoxin genes, and 5 enterotoxin genes. It also contains a novel gene cluster-*bsa* (bacteriocin of *S. aureus*) encodes a potential bacteriocin which increases the ability of colonization and chances of infection in the host (Baba et al., 2002; Gordon and Lowry 2008).

The strain USA300 and ST8 was responsible for causing rapid MRSA infections among prisoners, military personnel, athletes, and football players. The infections from this strain were reported internationally (Lina et al., 1999; Vandenesh et al., 2003). It was found to be becoming resistant to several non-β-lactam antibiotics (Diep et al., 2006). The whole genome sequencing of strain was performed and compared with previously isolated staphylococcal strains and the strain USA300 was found to be closely related to staphylococcal enterotoxins Q and K. It also possesses the bacteriocin gene cluster responsible for high virulence in this strain. The Arginine catabolic mobile element (ACME) was found in the USA300 strain which encodes an arginine deaminase pathway that converts L-arginine to carbon dioxide, adenosine triphosphate, and ammonia. ACME increases the virulence factor of this strain by enabling it to colonize the skin, open wound infections, and person to person contact.

The spread of CA-MRSA infections by genotypically variant MRSA strains was prevalent in other countries, such as ST93 strain in Australia, ST80 in European countries, ST59 in Asian countries, especially in Taiwan. It was also becoming increasingly resistant to non-β-lactam antibiotics (Tristan et al., 2007; Gould et al., 2012). The increased virulence in CA-MRSA strains is not completely understood, but the presence of the PVL gene in these strains with leukocytolytic activity enhances the virulence. A study conducted in France on 593 staphylococcal isolates revealed the presence of the PVL gene in CA-MRSA when compared to HA-MRSA (Dofour et al., 2002). PVL is an exotoxin and contains LukS-PV and LukF-PV subunits which together form pores in the cell and result in leukocyte destruction, such as neutrophils to release inflammatory enzymes and cytokines.

The PVL genes were found in almost 85% of community acquired pneumonia when compared with hospital associated MRSA infections. A study conducted by Lina et al. (2002) on 172 *Staphylococcus aureus* strains determined the presence of lukS-PV and lukF-PV subunits. PVL is not significantly associated with strains causing endocarditis, urinary tract infections, and toxic shock syndrome, but is significantly associated with skin or soft tissue infections and necrotizing pneumonia which enhances the virulence of CA-MRSA. The particular role of PVL in virulence of staphylococcal isolates and their establishment across the globe remains unclear and uncertain.

CA-MRSA can be prevented by maintaining necessary personal hygiene and cleanliness in the surroundings. Washing and sanitizing hands regularly should be adopted by all the individuals while using public areas. Healthcare workers or other employees in working areas should avoid open wounds, and workers with active infections should be excluded from work places, because skin-skin transmission is a major risk factor for MRSA spread among the community. The laundry material of an infected person should be washed properly with disinfectants or it should be decontaminated to avoid spread of infection. Decolonization of non-surgical wounds is also preferred to restrict the transmission of MRSA clones, one should take care and maintain proper hygiene when trying to drain the boils as it can spread. Farm workers should also maintain hygienic practices such as washing hands and feet regularly with alcohol-based solutions in the farm as well after leaving the farm.

Signs and Symptoms of MRSA Infection

In humans, MRSA infections appear as a red bump, a swollen area which is warm to touch, and full of pus accompanied by fever as described by CDC. Within a few days, the bump or inflamed area swells up and transforms into pus filled boil which increases the body temperature (Catherine et al., 2011). In the recent years, there is a continuous increase in MRSA infections among the general population, especially CA-MRSA and livestock-associated MRSA (LA-MRSA) (CDC 2013, Ferguson et al., 2016; WHO 2018). The various factors responsible for transmission of MRSA clones are listed below:

- *Household pets:* The close contact between humans and animal species, especially household pets such as dogs and cats create an exchange of organisms between humans and animals. The studies suggest that almost 9% of dogs in veterinary clinics and 7.8% of dogs in rescue shelters were reported with MRSA infections (Loeffler et al., 2005, 2010). The concurrent colonization of individuals and household pets is a risk factor for MRSA infections because most infections in pets affect the skin and soft tissue. The USA100/CMRSA-2 clone which is associated with community infection spread was reported among pets in North America (Weese et al., 2006, 2007; Tenover et al., 2008). Another strain responsible for epidemic in the UK was EMRSA-15 and 16 which was found in both humans and pets (Loeffler et al., 2005, 2010). It has been reported that MRSA clones- USA500/CMRSA-5 and USA100/CMRSA-2 evolved sporadic infections from humans to horses and these have adapted their survival in horses (Walther et al., 2009; Dujikeren et al., 2010).

- *Livestock MRSA (LA-MRSA):* The emergence and dissemination of MRSA clones in animals such as pigs, cattle and poultry have increased the risk of interspecies transmission. CC398 MRSA strain which lost its virulence to cause human associated infections and got adapted to livestock. The colonization of MRSA strain CC398 was found in pigs (24-86%), cattle (31-37%), poultry farmers (9-37%) and almost 44% in European pig-farmers (Kadlec et al., 2012; Mohamed et al., 2012; Ballhausen et al., 2017; Goerge et al., 2017). An unexpectedly high rate (760 times) of MRSA infections were reported in Dutch pig-farmers, Netherlands who had been in contact with pigs in comparison to the general population (Voss et al., 2005). ST398 strains have been reported to cause MRSA infections in pigs and also increases the possibility of dissemination of these clones to other species. Other human community epidemic strains USA100/CMRSA-2 were reported in pigs in Canada and ST9 in China (Khanna et al., 2007; Cui et al., 2009). The subsequent studies clearly confirmed that MRSA in pigs is a risk factor for spread of MRSA infections and colonization (Lewis et al., 2008; Van Rijen et al., 2008). The studies suggest that almost 47% of meat and poultry products sold in the United states (2011) were contaminated with staphylococcal strains and 15-25% of these strains were resistant to antibiotics. In 2014, LA-MRSA was reported in animal products of the UK, including milk tanks and retail meat, suggesting contamination from human sources during processing (Dhup et al., 2015; Sharma et al., 2016). The common MRSA strains isolated to cause infection in livestock are listed in Table 2.
  - Veterinary personnel are at high risk of acquiring LA-MRSA infections. There are several reports which indicate a high colonization rate in veterinary personnel due to occupational exposure. ST398 strains have been reported with 12.5% prevalence rate in swine veterinary attendees in the Netherlands (Wulf et al., 2007). The MRSA clones were predominantly reported in small animal veterinary staff (18%), veterinary

surgical attendees (17%), and veterinary technicians (12%) (Hanselman et al., 2006).

- The workers in animal husbandries, due to their occupational contact, become carriers of staphylococcal infections/resistance genes and transfer them to their family members (Nadimpalli et al., 2018). A study conducted on identification of MRSA strains in the indoor air of husbandries and also in fodder prepared for animals in 2016 revealed the prevalence of MRSA strains in smaller (5 µm) and larger particles (215 µm) (Ferguson et al., 2016). Another study was carried out to identify and confirm the presence and transmission of *S. aureus* through bioaerosols in poultry farms. The molecular methods applied in this study demonstrated the 60% similarity of isolated strains to *Staphylococcus aureus* suggesting the dissemination of MRSA clones from manure to farm workers (Zhong et al., 2009).
- Veterinary personnel and farmers working in animal farms are at high risk of developing infections caused by LA-MRSA, such as external otitis-common in swine farmers, accesses (fingers or jaw), toe wounds, conjunctivitis, and lymph node infections.

- *Intensive care units (ICUs):* The transmission of staphylococcal infections and prevalence of MRSA infections is higher in ICUs, especially surgical ICUs. These infections are highly associated with health care workers (HCW) and transmitted through hand-touched contaminated surfaces (Kei and Richard 2011). The factors increasing the chances of transmission are close skin-to-skin contact, catheters, open wounds, and poor personal hygiene. Airborne transmission is a direct transmission of MRSA clones through hands or mouth is also a concern (Chang and Lin 2018). The pathogenic strains of *Staphylococcus aureus* are able to survive under unfavourable conditions, like dry surfaces over a long period of time, and can be contagious when exposed to a host (Kramer et al., 2006; Boyce 2007; Hubner et al., 2011).

- *Public areas:* Children and athletes are prone to MRSA infections mainly from hospital acquired nurseries, day care centres, classroom, locker rooms, and playgrounds (Gopal and Divya 2017). The transmission of MRSA in skin or soft tissue injury is common through the use of towels, equipment, football playground turf, razors, and sharing personal items.
- *Waste-water treatment plants (WWTP):* The waste-water treatment plants are also an underlying factor for MRSA infections spread in communities. In 2012, samples were collected from four different wastewater treatment plants in the USA in order to analyse the bacteria inhabiting these plants. The samples were found to be 50% MRSA and 55% MSSA strains (Goldstein et al., 2012). In another study conducted by Thompson et al., (2013), MRSA strains in wastewater treatment plants originated from hospitals and could survive all the stages of treatment. The waste water treatment process generates enormous amounts of bioaerosols, which are directly or indirectly inhaled by treatment plant workers, causing colonization of MRSA clones in the respiratory tract (Bos et al., 2016).

The other risk factors responsible for MRSA outbreaks in communities, animal husbandries, or hospital settings include the transmission of pathogenic strains is listed in Table 3 (Mehta et al., 2020).

The risk factors mentioned in Table 3 increases the prevalence of MRSA clones within the community of healthy people which can be avoided to a certain level by following hygiene. The CDC suggests maintaining personal hygiene to avoid MRSA community outbreaks by washing hands regularly with soap or alcohol-based sanitizer. The regular screening of MRSA strains in hospital settings will also restrict the spread of HA-MRSA to CA-MRSA.

Table 2. Livestock associated-methicillin resistant strains in animal food

Sl. No.	MRSA clones	Animal source	References
1	CC130, ST395, ST425	Cattle, Dairy farms	Paterson et al., 2014
2	ST398	Swine/swine farm personnel	Hartley et al., 2014
3	CC9, CC22	Pig, chicken, beef	Dhup et al., 2015
4	ST398	Pork/swine, chicken	Hadjirin et al., 2015
5	CC398	Horses	Bortolami et al., 2017
6	ST398	Turkey, chicken and pig	Fox et al., 2017
7	CC398	Veal calf	Stone 2017
8	CC9/CC398	Turkey	Sharma et al., 2018

*Note: these strains have been isolated from various farms in Netherlands, Korea, United Kingdom, China, Switzerland, Malaysia and India.

Table 3. Risk factors associated for spread of methicillin-resistance *Staphylococcus aureus* infections

Sl. No.	Risk factors for MRSA infections
1	Individuals with longer stay in ICU's or hospital wards
2	Patients regularly visiting hospital for antimicrobial therapy or chemotherapy
3	Individuals with immunocompromised system
4	Patients with organ transplants
5	Regular drug users through syringes
6	HIV patients
7	Patients with chronic illness
8	Infants and elderly people
9	Diabetic patients
10	Patients with skin trauma-burns, cuts or sores
11	Individuals with skin tattoos or body piercin
12	Patients with open wounds in hospital wards.
13	Chronic obstructive pulmonary disease (COPD- patients)
14	Individuals ingesting unpasteurized milk
15	Veterinarians, pet holders and animal farmers

Treatment

The rapid increase in emergence of MRSA infections in community and hospital settings allows clinicians to change antibiotic prescription patterns which further increases the risk of antimicrobial resistance among MRSA strains. It was found that in developing countries the percentage of multidrug-resistant strains (MDR) among MRSA is very high, almost 73% (Arora et al., 2010). In 2017, WHO declared *Staphylococcus aureus* infections, methicillin resistant and vancomycin-resistant is a high threat to human health. The term methicillin-resistance refers to the ability of Staphylococcus (particularly MRSA) to resist the action of beta-lactam antibiotics. Over the last 40 years, staphylococcal strains acquiring resistance to β-lactam antibiotics has plagued the antimicrobial therapy (John 2020).

MRSA infections can be fatal, and delays in the treatment can claim many lives. Effective antibiotics against these infections can be introduced to patients intravenously or orally. Although staphylococcal strains conferred resistance to beta-lactam groups of antibiotics, vancomycin still remains to be the drug of choice to treat resistance infections (Catherine et al., 2011; John 2020). The synergistic effects of vancomycin and beta-lactam antibiotics have been found to act against resistant staphylococcal strains (Winn 2006). When MRSA appeared in the 1960's, the early strains contained a complex SCC*mec,* as well as multiple resistance genes. Vancomycin was one of the antibiotics to which MRSA strains were susceptible. Over the period of time, SCC*mec* evolved into many staphylococcal subtypes with antimicrobial resistance genes resulting in new strains of MRSA, and have been named vancomycin- intermediate resistant *Staphylococcus aureus* (VISA). Today, vancomycin is only used in initial therapy and remains the standard care treatment of resistant staphylococcal infections. The only drawback associated with vancomycin therapy is renal dysfunction (Sieradzki and Tomasz 1997; Schito 2006).

The traditional β-lactam antibiotics such as cephalexin which can treat a number of bacterial infections were found to be ineffective against emerging CA-MRSA and HA-MRSA strains. The introduction of sulpha drugs including trimethoprim, tetracycline, clindamycin and linezolid were reported to combat CA-MRSA infections up to 87%, reducing the risk for MRSA spread in community (Catherine et al., 2011; Guruswamy 2013).

The older and new antimicrobial agents to treat MRSA infections which can be used as an alternative to vancomycin are listed below:

- *Linezolid (brand name Zyvox):* an effective antibiotic over vancomycin to treat skin and soft tissue infections, and has been in use for almost 20 years. Linezolid is a successful alternative to vancomycin because 99.9% susceptibility was reported in staphylococcal isolates whereas the percentage of successful vancomycin treatment is as low as 47% (Pfaller et al., 2017; Guruswamy 2013).
- *Daptomycin:* is a lipopeptide antibiotic effective against Gram positive bacteria that has become a good alternative to vancomycin. It has a bactericidal effect towards MRSA strains and has been approved to treat skin and soft tissue infections (SSTTIs), and acute bacterial skin and skin structure infections (ABSSSIs). It is not approved to treat pneumonia because the compound is highly bound to pulmonary surfactant (Baltz 2009, John 2020).
- *Ceftaroline:* Its brand name is Teflaro-a. Cephalosporin is an antibiotic which was avoided for years by clinicians to treat MRSA infections and is active against MRSA and other Gram positive bacterial infections. In 2010, FDA advisory committee approved ceftaroline for the treatment of community associated pneumonia and skin infections.
- *Fosfomycin:* brand name Monural-is a broad spectrum antibiotic effective against Gram positive and Gram negative pathogenic bacterial strains. This antibiotic is used against urinary tract infections (UTI) and given in combination with anti-staphylococcal agents (Jia 2018).
- *Oritavancin:* is a lipoglycopeptide structurally similar to vancomycin. It is effective against Gram positive infections. It has a long half-life and administered in patients through IV infusions

over the course of three hours. Dalbavancin also has extremely long half-life and patients are treated weekly for staphylococcal infections, especially methicillin-resistance *Staphylococcus epidermidis* (MRSE) and endocarditis (Tobudic et al., 2018).

- *Tigecycline:* It is a tetracycline derivative. It is a broad-spectrum antibiotic to treat skin abscesses and intra-abdominal infections caused by staphylococcal strains (Scheinfeld 2005). It is highly effective against MRSA biofilms, penetration into tissue and bone, infected wounds, and osteomyelitis (Griffin et al., 2013).
- *Televancin*: is a lipoglycopeptide used against MRSA and other Gram positive bacterial infections. In 2009, FDA approved this drug for the treatment of complicated skin and skin-structure infections (cSSSI), and hospital acquired staphylococcal pneumonia.
- *Combination therapy:* The combination therapy of antibiotics has been successful to combat MRSA infections in community as well as hospital settings. For example, daptomycin and ceftaroline, vancomycin and cefazolin, and daptomycin and beta-lactam antibiotics (Geriak et al., 2019; Trinh et al., 2017). Among all the antibiotics introduced in the last few decades, vancomycin and daptomycin remains the standard care therapy for resistance strains of Staphylococci.

CONCLUSION

The gradual increase in methicillin-resistant staphylococcal infections in community, hospitals, and livestock is alarming and is a major public health concern for several years. However, it is clear that MRSA infections affect both human and animal populations. A balanced approach is the key to reduce the manifestations of MRSA clones. The dissemination of MRSA clones from health care settings to community and animal population is the major risk factor for antimicrobial resistance in staphylococcal strains. Fighting against this transmission is challenging, but can be achieved by global public awareness, by reducing the use of antibiotics in animal food, isolating and decolonizing individuals, by promoting the development of therapeutics, and improved hygiene and precautionary measures. The infectious disease society of America has promoted the development of new agents with novel mechanisms of antibacterial and anti-staphylococcal activity. We must continue to fight against MRSA infections, which requires proper understanding and knowledge of the emergence and dissemination of MRSA strains in various regions. The combination therapies of old traditional drugs remain the mainstay for various staphylococcal infections in hospital and community settings, but the continuous increase in antimicrobial resistance will no longer sustain these therapies. Therefore, we must promote the development of new agents to combat the spread of MRSA infections.

REFERENCES

Amaral, M. M., Coelho, L. R., Flores, R. P. et al. (2005) The predominant variant of the Brazilian epidemic clonal complex of methicillin-resistant *Staphylococcus aureus* has an enhanced ability to produce biofilm and to adhere to and invade airway epithelial cells. *J Infect Dis*; 192:801–10.

Arora, S., Devi, P., Arora, U., Devi, B. (2010) Prevalence of methicillin-resistant *Staphylococcus aureus* (MRSA) in a Tertiary Care Hospital in Northern India. *J Lab Physicians*;278–81.

Baba, T., Takeuchi, F., Kuroda, M, Yuzawa, H., Aoki, K., Oguchi, A., Nagai, Y., Iwama, N., Asano, K., Naimi, T., Kuroda, H., Cui, L., Yamamoto, K., Hiramatsu, K. (2002) Genome and virulence determinants of high virulence community-acquired MRSA. *Lancet*: 359:1819–27.

Ballhausen, B., Kriegeskorte, A., van Alen S., Jung, P., Kock, R., Peters, G., et al. (2017). The pathogenicity and host adaptation of livestock-associated MRSA CC398. *Vet. Microbiol.* 200 39–45.

Baltz, R. H. (2009) Daptomycin: mechanisms of action and resistance, and biosynthetic engineering. *Current Opinion in Chemical Biology.* 13 (2): 144–51.

Berkley, S. F., Hightower, A. W., Broome, C. V., Reingold, A. L. The relationship of tampon characteristics to menstrual toxic shock syndrome. *JAMA* 1987, *258*, 917–920.

Bortolami, A., Williams, N. J., McGowan, C. M., Kelly, P. G., Archer, D. C., Corro, M., et al. (2017). Environmental surveillance identifies multiple introductions of MRSA CC398 in an equine veterinary hospital in the UK, 2011-2016. *Sci. Rep.* 7:5499.

Bos, ME., Verstappen, K. M, Cleef, B. A., Dohmen W et al. (2016) Transmission through air as a possible route of exposure for MRSA. J Expo Sci Environ Epidemiol 26(3):263–269.

Boyce, J. M. (2007) Environmental contamination makes an important contribution to hospital infection. *J Hosp Infect* 65:50–54.

Canadian Committee on Antibiotic Resistance. *Canadian Communicable Disease Report Antibiotic Resistance Issue September* (2003). Available at: http://www.ccarccra.com/english/pdfs/cdr2918.pdf.

Catry, B., Latour, K., Jans, B., Vandendriessche, S., Preal, R., Mertens K, et al. (2014) Risk factors for methicillin resistant *Staphylococcus aureus*: a multi-laboratory study. *PLoS One*;9:e89579.

Centers for Disease Control and Prevention (CDC) (2013) *Antibiotic resistance threats in the United States.* Atlanta: CDC; 2013.

Centers for Disease Control and Prevention. Four pediatric deaths from community-acquired methicillin-resistant *Staphylococcus aureus*— Minnesota and North Dakota, 1997-1999. *J Am Med Assoc* 1999; 282: 1123-1125.

Centers for Disease Control and Prevention. Four pediatric deaths from community-acquired methicillin-resistant *Staphylococcus aureus*— Minnesota and North Dakota, 1997–1999. *JAMA* 1999; 282:1123–5.

Centers for Disease Control and Prevention. *Methicillin-resistant Staphylococcus aureus skin or soft=tissue infections in a state prison—* Mississippi, 2000. MMWR 2001; 50: 919-922.

Chambers, H. F., DeLeo, F. R. (2009) Waves of resistance: *Staphylococcus aureus* in the antibiotic era. *Nat Rev Microbiol* 7:629-641.

Chang, C. W., Lin, M. H. (2018) Optimization of PMA-qPCR for *Staphylococcus aureus* and determination of viable bacteria in indoor air. *Indoor Air*; 28:64–72.

Cui, S., Li, J., Hu, C., Jin, S., Li, F., Guo, Y., Ran, L., Ma, Y. (2009) Isolation and characterization of methicillin-resistant *Staphylococcus aureus* from swine and workers in China. *J Antimicrob Chemother* 64:680-683.

Daum, R. S. (2007) Skin and Soft-Tissue infections caused by Methicillin-Resistant *Staphylococcus aureus*. *New England Journal of Medicine*. 357 (4): 380–390.

Dhup V., Kearns A. M., Pichon B., Foster H. A. (2015). First report of identification of livestock-associated MRSA ST9 in retail meat in England. *Epidemiol. Infect.* 143 2989–2992.

Diep, B. A., Gill, S. R., Chang, R. F., et al. (2006). Complete genome sequence of USA300, an epidemic clone of community-acquired methicillin-resistant *Staphylococcus aureus*. *Lancet*; 367:731–9.

Donlan, R. M., Costerton, J. W. (2002) Biofilms: survival mechanisms of clinically relevant microorganisms. *Clin Microbiol Rev*; 15:167–93.

Dufour, P., Gillet, Y., Bes M, et al. (2002) Community-acquired methicillin-resistant *Staphylococcus aureus* infections in France: emergence of a single clone that produces Panton-Valentine leukocidin. *Clin Infect Dis*; 35:819–24.

Eckhardt, C., Halvosa, J. S., Ray, S. M., Blumberg, H. M. (2003) Transmission of methicillin-resistant *Staphylococcus aureus* in the neonatal intensive care unit from a patient with community-acquired disease. *Infect Control Hosp Epidemiol*; 24: 460- 461.

Ferguson, D., Smith, T., Hanson, B., Wardyn, S., Donham, K. (2016) Detection of airborne methicillin – resistant *Staphylococcus aureus* inside and downwind of a swine building, and in animal feed: potential occupational, animal health, and environmental implications. *J Agromedicine*; 21(2):149–153.

Foster, T. J., Hook, M. (1998) Surface protein adhesins of *Staphylococcus aureus*. *Trends Microbiol*; 6:484– 8.

Four pediatric deaths from community-acquired methicillin-resistant *Staphylococcus aureus*— Minnesota and North Dakota, 1997–1999. MMWR Morb Mortal Wkly Rep 1999; 48:707–10.

Fox, A., Pichon, B., Wilkinson, H., Doumith, M., Hill, R. L. R., McLauchlin J., et al. (2017). Detection and molecular characterization of livestock-associated MRSA in raw meat on retail sale in North West England. *Lett. Appl. Microbiol.* 64 239–245.

Geriak, M., Haddad, F., Rizvi, K., et al. (2019) Clinical data on Daptomycin plus Ceftaroline versus standard of care monotherapy in the treatment of Methicillin-Resistant *Staphylococcus aureus* bacteremia. *Antimicrob Agents Chemother*; 63(5):pii: e02483-18.

Goerge, T., Lorenz, M. B., van Alen S., Hubner, N. O., Becker, K., Kock, R. (2017). MRSA colonization and infection among persons with occupational livestock exposure in Europe: prevalence, preventive options and evidence. *Vet. Microbiol.* 200 6–12.

Gopal, S., Divya, K. C. (2017). Can methicillin-resistant *Staphylococcus aureus* prevalence from dairy cows in India act as potential risk for community-associated infections? A review. *Veterinary World.* 10: 311–318.

Gordon, Y. C., Amer E. V., Hwang-Soo, J., Anthony D. C., Anthony, J. Y., Thuan H. N., Daniel, E. S., Queck S. Y., Otto, M. (2014) Genome-wide analysis of the regulatory function mediated by the small regulatory psm-mec RNA of methicillin-resistant *Staphylococcus aureus*. *International Journal of Medical Microbiology*; 304: 637–644.

Gould, I. M., David, M. Z., Esposito, S., Garau, J., Lina, G., Mazzei, T., Peters, G. (2012). "New insights into meticillin-resistant *Staphylococcus aureus* (MRSA) pathogenesis, treatment and resistance." *Int. J. Antimicrob. Agents* (2): 96–104.

Griffin, A. T., Harting, J. A., Christensen, D. M. (2013). Tigecycline in the management of osteomyelitis: a case series from the bone and joint infection (BAJIO) database. *Diagn Microbiol Infect Dis*;77(3):273–7.

Hadjirin, N. F., Lay, E. M., Paterson, G. K., Harrison, E. M., Peacock, S. J., Parkhill, J., et al. (2015). Detection of livestock-associated meticillin-resistant *Staphylococcus aureus* CC398 in retail pork, United Kingdom, February 2015. *Eurosurveillance* 20 1–4.

Hanselman, B., Kruth, S., Rousseau, J., Low, D., Willey, B., McGeer, A., Weese, J. (2006) Methicillin-resistant *Staphylococcus aureus* colonization in veterinary personnel. *Emerg Infect Dis*: 12:1933-1938.

Hartley, H., Watson, C., Nugent, P., Beggs, N., Dickson, E., Kearns, A. (2014). Confirmation of LA-MRSA in pigs in the UK. *Vet. Rec.* 175 74–75.

Herold, B. C., Immergluck, L. C., Maranan, M. C., Lauderdale, D. S., Gaskin, R. E., Boyle-Vavra S, et al. (1998) Community-acquired methicillin-resistant *Staphylococcus aureus* in children with no identified predisposing risk. *JAMA;* 279: 593-598.

Hubner, N. O., Hubner, C., Kramer. A., Assadian, O. (2011) Survival of bacterial pathogens on paper and bacterial retrieval from paper to hands: preliminary results. *Am J Nurs*; 111:30–34.

Ito, T., Ma, X. X., Takeuchi, F., Okuma, K., Yuzawa, H., Hiramatsu, K (2004) Novel type V staphylococcal cassette chromosome mec driven by a novel cassette chromosome recombinase, ccrC. *Antimicrob Agents Che-mother*; 48:2637–51.

Jensen, S. O., Lyon, B. R. (2009) Genetics of antimicrobial resistance in *Staphylococcus aureus*. *Future Microbiol.* 4 (5): 565–82.

Jia, Y. (2018). The progress in study of fosfomycin. *Infection International*; 6(3):88–92.

Kadlec, K., Fessler, A. T., Hauschild, T., Schwarz, S. (2012). Novel and uncommon antimicrobial resistance genes in livestock-associated methicillin-resistant *Staphylococcus aureus*. *Clin. Microbiol. Infect.* 18 745–755.

Kallen, A. J., Driscoll, T. J., Thornton, S., Olson, P. E., Wallace, M. R. (2000) Increase in community-acquired methicillin-resistant *Staphylococcus aureus* at a Naval Medical Center. *Infect Control Hosp Epidemiol*; 21: 223-226.

Kazakova, S. V., Hageman, J. C., Matava, M., Srinivasan, A., Phelan, L., Garfinkel B, et al. (2005) A clone of methicillin-resistant

Staphylococcus aureus among professional football players. *N Engl J Med*; 352: 468-475.

Kei, J., Richards, J. R. (2011). The prevalence of methicillin-resistant *Staphylococcus aureus* on inanimate objects in an urban emergency department. *J Emerg Med*;41(2):124–127.

Khanna, T., Friendship, R., Dewey, C., Weese, J. S. (2007). Methicillin resistant *Staphylococcus aureus* colonization in pigs and pig farmers. *Vet Microbiol* 128:298-303.

Klevens, R. M., Edwards, J. R., Tenover, F. C., McDonald, L. C., Horan, T., Gaynes, R. (2006). Changes in the epidemiology of methicillin-resistant *Staphylococcus aureus* in intensive care units in US hospitals, 1992–2003. *Clin Infect Dis*; 42:389–91.

Kluytmans, J., Belkum V. A, Verbrugh, H. (1997). Nasal carriage of *Staphylococcus aureus*: epidemiology, underlying mechanisms, and associated risks. *Clin Microbiol Rev*; 10:505–20.

Kong, C., Neoh, H., Nathan, S. (2016). Targetting *Staphylococcus aureus* toxins: A potential form of anti-virulence therapy. *Toxins*; 8:72.

Kozajda, A., Jeżak, K., Kapsa, A. (2019). Airborne *Staphylococcus aureus* in different environments—a review. *Environ Sci Pollut Res* 26, 34741–34753.

Kramer, A., Schwebke, I., Kampf, G. (2006). How long do nosocomial pathogens persist on inanimate surfaces? A systematic review. *BMC Infect Dis* 16(6):130.

Kuehnert, M. J., Hill, H. A., Kupronis, B. A., Tokars, J. I., Solomon, S. L., Jernigan, D. B. (2005). Methicillin-resistant–*Staphylococcus aureus* hospitalizations, United States. *Emerg Infect Dis*; 11:868–72.

Lina, G., Piemont, Y., Godail-Gamot F, et al. Involvement of Panton-Valentine leukocidin–producing *Staphylococcus aureus* in primary skin infections and pneumonia. *Clin Infect Dis* 1999;29:1128–32.

Liu, C., Bayer, A., Cosgrove, S. E., Daum, R. S., Fridkin, S. K., Gorwitz, R. J., Kaplan, S. L., Karchmer, A. W., Levine, D. P., Murray, B. E., Rybak, J. M., Talan, D. A., Chambers, H. F. (2011). Clinical practice guidelines by the Infectious Diseases society of America for the treatment of

Methicillin-Resistant *Staphylococcus aureus* Infections in Adults and Children. *Clinical Infectious Diseases*; 53(3):319.

Loeffler, A., Boag, A., Sung, J., Lindsay, J., Guardabassi, L., Dalsgaard, A., Smith, H., Stevens, K., Lloyd, D. (2005). Prevalence of methicillin-resistant *Staphylococcus aureus* among staff and pets in a small animal referral hospital in the UK. *J Antimicrob Chemother*; 56:692-697.

Loeffler, A., Pfeiffer, D. U., Lindsay, J. A., Soares-Magalhaes, R., Lloyd, D. H. (2010). Lack of transmission of methicillin-resistant *Staphylococcus aureus* (MRSA) between apparently healthy dogs in a rescue kennel. *Vet Microbiol*; 141:178-181.

Lowy, F. D. (1998). *Staphylococcus aureus* infections. *N Engl J Med*; 339(8):520-32.

Mehta, Y., Hegde, A., Pande, R. et al. (2020). Methicillin-resistant *Staphylococcus aureus* in Intensive Care Unit Setting of India: A Review of Clinical Burden, Patterns of Prevalence, Preventive Measures, and Future Strategies. *Indian J Crit Care Med*; 24(1):55–62.

Melter, O., Radojevic, B. (2010). Small colony variants of *Staphylococcus aureus*--review. *Folia Microbiol* (Praha); 55(6):548-58.

Mohamed, D. H., Saberesheikh, S., Kearns, A. M., Saunders, N. A. (2012). Putative link between *Staphylococcus aureus* bacteriophage serotype and community association. *Int. J. Med. Microbiol.* 302 135–144.

Murray, Patrick (2007). *Manual of clinical microbiology*. Washington, D.C: ASM Press. ISBN 978-1-55581-371-0.

Nadimpalli, M. L., Stewart, J. R., Pierce, E., Pisanic, N., Love, D. C., Hall, D., Larsen, J., Carroll, K. C., Tekle, T., Perl, T. M., Heaney, C. D. (2018). Face mask use and persistence of livestock-associated *Staphylococcus aureus* nasal carriage among industrial hog operation workers and household contacts, USA. *Environ Health Perspect*; 126(12):127005.

National Nosocomial Infections Surveillance System. National Nosocomial Infections Surveillance (NNIS) System report, data summary from January 1992 through June 2004, issued October 2004. *Am J Infect Control* 2004; 32:470–85.

New Drug Approvals. 29 October 2010. Retrieved 8 November 2010.

Noskin, G. A., Rubin, R. J., Schentag, J. J., Kluytmans, J., Hedblom, E. C., Smulders, M. et al. (2005). The burden of *Staphylococcus aureus* infections on hospitals in the United States: an analysis of the 2000 and 2001 nationwide inpatient sample database. *Arch Intern Med*; 165:1756–61.

Paterson, G. K., Morgan, F. J., Harrison, E. M., Peacock, S. J., Parkhill, J., Zadoks, R. N., et al. (2014). Prevalence and properties of mecC methicillin-resistant *Staphylococcus aureus* (MRSA) in bovine bulk tank milk in Great Britain. *J Antimicrob Chemother* 69 598–602.

Patti, J. M., Allen, B. L., McGavin, M. J., Hook, M. (1994) MSCRAMM-mediated adherence of microorganisms to host tissues. *Annu Rev Microbiol*; 48:585–617.

Pfaller, M. A., Mendes, R. E., Streit, J. M., et al. (2011-2015). Five-Year Summary of *In Vitro* Activity and Resistance Mechanisms of Linezolid against Clinically Important Gram-Positive Cocci in the United States from the LEADER Surveillance Program (2011 to 2015). *Antimicrob Agents Chemother.* 2017;61(7): pii: e00609-17.

Rosenberg Goldstein, R. E., Micallef, S. A., Gibbs, S. G., Davis, J. A. et al. (2012). Methicillin – resistant *Staphylococcus aureus* (MRSA) detected at four U.S. wastewater treatment plants. *Environ Health Perspect*; 120(11):1551–1558.

Scheinfeld, N (2005). Tigecycline: a review of a new glycylcycline antibiotic *Journal of Dermatological Treatment*; 16 (4): 207–12.

Schito, G. C. (2006). The importance of the development of antibiotic resistance in *Staphylococcus aureus*. *Clin Microbiol Infect*. 12 (Suppl 1): 3–8.

Selvan, G. K., Peter, W., Brian, R. D. (2013). Gurusamy, Kurinchi Selvan (ed.). "Antibiotic therapy for the treatment of methicillin-resistant *Staphylococcus aureus* (MRSA) in non-surgical wounds." *Cochrane Database of Systematic Reviews*.

Sharma M., Nunez-Garcia J., Kearns A. M., Doumith M., Butaye P. R., Angeles Argudín M., et al. (2016). Livestock-associated methicillin resistant *Staphylococcus aureus* (LA-MRSA) clonal complex (CC) 398 isolated from UK animals belong to European lineages. *Front. Microbiol.* 7:1741.

Sieradzki, K., Tomasz, A. (1997). Inhibition of cell wall turnover and autolysis by vancomycin in a highly vancomycin-resistant mutant of *Staphylococcus aureus*. *J. Bacteriol.* 179 (8): 2557–66.

Stone, K. (2017). Risk Assessment on Meticillin-Resistant *Staphylococcus aureus* (MRSA), with a focus on Livestock-associated MRSA, in the UK *Food Chain*. London: Food Standard Agency.

Tenover, F. C., McAllister, S., Fosheim, G., McDougal, L. K., Carey, R. B., Limbago, B., Lonsway, D., Patel, J. B., Kuehnert, M. J., Gorwitz, R. (2008). Characterization of *Staphylococcus aureus* isolates from nasal cultures collected from individuals in the United States in 2001 to 2004. *J Clin Microbiol*; 46:2837-2841.

Thompson, J. M., Gundogdu, A., Stratton, H. M., Katouli, M. (2013). Antibiotic resistant *Staphylococcus aureus* in hospital wastewaters and sewage treatment plants with special reference to methicillin – resistant *Staphylococcus aureus* (MRSA). *J Appl Microbiol*; 114(1):44–54.

Tobudic, S., Forstner, C., Burgmann, H., et al. (2018). Dalbavancin as Primary and Sequential Treatment for Gram-Positive Infective Endocarditis: 2-Year Experience at the General Hospital of Vienna. *Clin Infect Dis*; 67(5):795–8.

Trinh, T. D., Zasowski, E. J., Lagnf, A. M. et al. (2017). Combination Vancomycin/Cefazolin (VAN/CFZ) for Methicillin-Resistant *Staphylococcus aureus* (MRSA) Bloodstream Infections (BSI). *Open Forum Infect Dis.* 2017;4(Supp 1): S281.

Tristan, A., Bes, M., Meugnier, H., Lina, G., Bozdogan, B., Courvalin, P., Reverdy, M. E., Enright, M. C., Vandenesch, F., Etienne, J. (2007). Global distribution of Panton–Valentine leukocidin--positive methicillin-resistant *Staphylococcus aureus*, 2006. *Emerg Infect Dis;* 13(4):594-600.

Tung, H., Guss, B., Hellman, U., Persson, L., Rubin, K., Ryden, C. (2000). A bone sialoprotein-binding protein from *Staphylococcus aureus*: a member of the staphylococcal Sdr family. *Biochem J*; 345:611–9.

Udo, E. E., Pearman, J. W., Grubb, W. B. (1993). Genetic analysis of community isolates of methicillin-resistant *Staphylococcus aureus* in western Australia. *J Hosp Infect*; 25:97–108.

Vandenesch, F., Lina, G., Henry, T. *Staphylococcus aureus* hemolysins, bi-component leukocidins, and cytolytic peptides: A redundant arsenal of membrane-damaging virulence factors? *Front. Cell. Infect. Microbiol.* 2012, *2*, 12.

Vandenesch, F., Naimi, T., Enright, M. C., et al. (2003). Community-acquired methicillin-resistant *Staphylococcus aureus* carrying Panton-Valentine leukocidin genes: worldwide emergence. *Emerg Infect Dis*; 9:978–84.

Voss, A., Loeffen, F., Bakker, J., Klaassen, C., Wulf, M. (2005). Methicillin resistant *Staphylococcus aureus* in pig farming. *Emerging Infect Dis:* 11:1965-1966.

Walev, I., Weller, U., Strauch, S., Foster, T., Bhakdi, S. Selective killing of human monocytes and cytokine release provoked by sphingomyelinase (beta-toxin) of *Staphylococcus aureus. Infect. Immun.* 1996, *64*, 2974–2979.

Walther, B., Monecke, S., Ruscher, C., Friedrich, A. W., Ehricht, R., Slickers, P., Soba, A., Wleklinski, C. G., Wieler, L. H., Lübke-Becker A. (2009). Comparative molecular analysis substantiates zoonotic potential of equine methicillinresistant *Staphylococcus aureus. J Clin Microbiol*; 47:704-710.

Weese, J., Dick, H., Willey, B., McGeer, A., Kreiswirth, B., Innis, B., Low, D. (2006b). Suspected transmission of methicillin-resistant *Staphylococcus aureus* between domestic pets and humans in veterinary clinics and in the household. *Vet Microbiol*; 115:148-155.

Weese, J. S., Faires, M., Rousseau, J., Bersenas, A. M., Mathews, K. A. (2007). Cluster of methicillin-resistant *Staphylococcus aureus* colonization in a small animal intensive care unit. *JAVMA*; 231:1361-1364.

Wertheim, H. F., Melles, D. C., Vos, M. C., et al. (2005). The role of nasal carriage in *Staphylococcus aureus* infections. *Lancet Infect Dis*; 5:751–62.

Wilke, G. A., Bubeck Wardenburg, J. (2010). Role of a disintegrin and metalloprotease 10 in *Staphylococcus aureus* alpha-hemolysin-mediated cellular injury. *Proc. Natl. Acad. Sci. USA*; 107 13473–13478.

Winn, Washington (2006). *Koneman's color atlas and textbook of diagnostic microbiology*. Philadelphia: Lippincott Williams & Wilkins. ISBN 978-0-7817-3014-3.

World Health Organization (2018). Global antimicrobial resistance surveillance system (GLASS) report: early implementation 2016-2017.

Wu, S. W., Lencastre, H. (2001). "Recruitment of the mecA gene homolog of Staphyoloccus sciuri into a resistance determinant and expression of the resistance phenotype in *Staphylococcus aureus*." *Journal of Bacteriology*; 183 (8): 2417–24.

Wulf, M. W., Sorum, M., Nes, A., Skov, R., Melchers, W. J., Klaassen, C. H., Voss, A. (2007). Prevalence of methicillin-resistant *Staphylococcus aureus* among veterinarians: An international study. *Clin Microbiol Infect*; 14:519-521.

Zetola, N., Francis, J. S., Nuermberger, E. L., Bishai, W. R. (2005). Community-acquired methicillin-resistant *Staphylococcus aureus*: an emerging threat. *Lancet Infect Dis*; 5:275–86.

Zhong, Z., Chai, T., Duan, H., Li, X. et al. (2009). REP – PCR tracking of the origin and spread of airborne *Staphylococcus aureus* in and around chicken house. *Indoor Air* 19(6):511–516.

INDEX

A

acid, 6, 7, 11, 29, 32, 43, 99, 100, 101, 119, 126, 127, 143, 144, 146, 150, 152
acute glomerulonephritis, 125
acute infection, 80
adenosine triphosphate, 27, 164
adults, 11, 17, 18, 45, 51, 53, 54, 115, 125, 132, 134, 136, 137, 138, 142, 147, 151
adverse event, vii, 2, 5, 12
airway epithelial cells, 174
alternative medicine, 36, 39
alternative treatments, 6
antibiotic, vii, x, 2, 6, 9, 10, 11, 13, 24, 28, 30, 31, 35, 37, 38, 39, 44, 45, 62, 81, 85, 86, 88, 92, 93, 94, 97, 102, 104, 106, 108, 109, 110, 114, 115, 120, 122, 126, 129, 130, 133, 135, 136, 137, 151, 155, 156, 159, 161, 171, 172, 173, 176, 181
antibiotic resistance, x, 24, 39, 40, 41, 62, 81, 85, 88, 109, 114, 155, 156, 161, 175, 181
antibody, 9, 11, 19, 42, 44
antigen, 8, 9, 13, 14, 54
antimicrobial therapy, 170, 171
athletes, 157, 164, 169

B

bacteremia, ix, 4, 11, 13, 14, 16, 19, 20, 24, 46, 47, 49, 52, 56, 89, 90, 93, 95, 105, 110, 111, 112, 113, 118, 119, 121, 122, 129, 130, 131, 132, 137, 140, 141, 142, 143, 144, 145, 146, 147, 148, 149, 151, 152, 156, 162, 177
bacteria, viii, 2, 4, 5, 7, 9, 10, 19, 20, 21, 22, 23, 26, 27, 28, 29, 30, 34, 35, 36, 37, 38, 54, 62, 64, 68, 81, 83, 84, 90, 91, 93, 94, 96, 97, 98, 99, 100, 102, 103, 104, 113, 114, 128, 131, 137, 139, 140, 144, 148, 158, 159, 169, 172, 176
bacterial cells, 22, 103
bacterial infection, x, 3, 7, 24, 26, 29, 30, 33, 62, 100, 108, 115, 155, 171, 172, 173
bacterial pathogens, 80, 124, 178
bacterial strains, 172

bactericides, 104
bacteriophage, 7, 22, 24, 57, 58, 59, 82, 180
bacteriophages, iv, vii, 2, 3, 6, 7, 20, 21, 22, 23, 24, 25, 57, 58, 60
bacteriostatic, 7, 97, 135
bacterium, 4, 5, 7, 8, 9, 10, 16, 34, 82, 85, 100, 122
bioavailability, 98
biocompatibility, 27, 99, 101
biological activities, 37
biological activity, 71
biological processes, 103
biological systems, 34
biomolecules, 25
biosynthesis, 87, 94
blood, 10, 11, 12, 21, 83, 130, 133, 135, 137, 159
blood cultures, 12
blood flow, 137
blood stream, 130
bloodstream, 47, 81, 110, 113
bone, 19, 93, 122, 130, 134, 135, 136, 138, 148, 150, 158, 173, 177, 182
bone and joint infections, 93, 122, 130, 148, 150, 158
botanical medicine, iv, vii, viii, 2, 3, 6, 36
Brazil, 1, 2, 43, 69, 70, 71, 72, 73, 74, 75, 79, 108, 119, 162

C

cardiac surgery, 137
catheter, 87, 130, 131, 158
cefazolin, 101, 109, 173
ceftaroline, 87, 95, 105, 118, 129, 132, 133, 141, 172, 173, 177
cell culture, 10
cell death, viii, 3, 27, 28, 91, 93, 123, 124, 160
cell division, 103
cell membranes, 28
cell surface, 8, 21
cellulitis, 127, 128, 143, 146, 147, 150
central nervous system, 137
challenges, 20, 37, 49, 109, 114, 131, 145
chemical, 33, 96, 98, 101
chemical stability, 101
chemiluminescence, 28
chemotherapy, x, 47, 58, 112, 156, 170
children, 115, 125, 126, 134, 136, 143, 147, 157, 178
chitosan, 29, 100, 101, 107, 116
chromosome, ix, 21, 86, 121, 123, 151, 161, 178
chronic obstructive pulmonary disease, 133
classes, 81, 92, 104, 106, 123
clindamycin, 81, 84, 122, 126, 128, 135, 146, 147, 172
clinical application, 23, 63
clinical presentation, 125, 135
clinical symptoms, 136
clinical trials, viii, 2, 10, 13, 15, 19, 20, 50
clone, 8, 25, 105, 130, 161, 162, 166, 176, 178
colonization, 5, 20, 55, 56, 83, 88, 108, 113, 117, 134, 158, 160, 164, 166, 167, 169, 177, 178, 179, 183
combination therapy, 95, 106, 173
combined therapy, 13, 94
community-associated (CA-MRSA), 81, 87, 88, 111, 123, 124, 130, 157, 159, 163, 165, 166, 169, 171
complications, 13, 20, 85, 126, 128, 130, 135
composition, 26, 76, 97
compounds, viii, 2, 26, 33, 37, 81, 92, 99, 102
contaminated food, 159
contamination, 167, 175
culture, 12, 35, 87, 130, 136, 139
culture media, 136
cure, 13, 33, 34
cystic fibrosis, 11, 159

cytokines, 34, 97, 160, 165
cytoplasm, viii, 2, 23, 33

D

daptomycin, 84, 90, 93, 95, 104, 105, 110, 114, 118, 120, 129, 131, 132, 137, 140, 142, 144, 147, 151, 172, 173, 175, 177
database, 3, 177, 181
deaths, 4, 175, 177
debridement, 60, 135
decolonization, 162
dermatology, 143, 150, 152
destruction, 5, 28, 36, 134, 165
detection, 62, 83, 115
developing countries, 171
diabetic patients, 29
disease progression, 10, 45
diseases, 3, 4, 8, 33, 36, 80, 90, 115, 125, 136, 147, 150, 159, 160
diversity, 22, 83, 123
DNA, 5, 20, 21, 23, 28, 31, 32, 36, 37, 68
drug delivery, 25, 28, 116
drug release, 26
drug resistance, 98
drugs, viii, x, 2, 4, 8, 10, 25, 33, 35, 37, 38, 81, 82, 87, 88, 92, 94, 95, 104, 105, 106, 109, 122, 128, 138, 139, 155, 172, 174

E

electromagnetic, 34
electromagnetic fields, 34
electromagnetic waves, 34
encapsulation, 25, 27, 82, 95, 99, 101, 106
environment, 4, 5, 22, 37, 80, 82, 84, 88, 100, 102, 134
enzymatic activity, 36
enzymes, 37, 75, 83, 159, 165
epidemic, 110, 162, 166, 167, 174, 176
epidemiology, ix, 80, 84, 109, 110, 113, 114, 139, 149, 151, 179
evidence, 5, 40, 104, 119, 177
exposure, 133, 137, 157, 167, 175, 177
extracellular matrix, 5, 84, 137
extracts, viii, 2, 36, 37, 38, 40, 67, 71, 97, 98, 102, 104, 107
exudate, 125, 128

F

family members, 162, 168
farmers, 88, 167, 168, 170, 179
fermentation, 75, 76, 82
fever, 91, 130, 166
food, 65, 75, 76, 83, 98, 105, 159, 160, 170, 173
food additive, 105
Food and Drug Administration (FDA), 20, 99, 105, 111, 126, 172, 173
food poisoning, 83, 159
food products, 159
football, 164, 169, 179
fusidic acid, 100, 119, 126, 127, 143, 144, 146, 150, 152
fusion, 8, 9, 16, 52

G

gene expression, 103
gene transfer, 23, 161
genes, 5, 21, 23, 56, 89, 161, 164, 165, 168, 171, 178, 183
genetic diversity, 118
genetic engineering, 22
genetic information, 21
genome, 20, 21, 22, 164, 176
growth, viii, 3, 7, 26, 27, 31, 34, 36, 37, 44, 94, 100, 104
growth rate, viii, 3
guidelines, 115, 147, 179

H

half-life, 12, 45, 102, 172
healing, 7, 29, 32, 33, 102
health, x, 3, 7, 31, 33, 37, 69, 72, 81, 87, 123, 155, 157, 162, 163, 168, 173, 176
health care, x, 123, 155, 157, 163, 168, 173
health care system, 157
health problems, 37
health services, 87
homeopathy, iv, vii, viii, 2, 3, 6, 7, 33, 34, 35, 43, 44, 65, 66, 71
hospital-associated (HA-MRSA), x, 81, 87, 88, 107, 111, 123, 155, 157, 161, 162, 163, 165, 169, 171
hospitalization, 19, 87, 128, 133, 135
host, 5, 8, 9, 10, 19, 20, 21, 22, 31, 34, 38, 51, 56, 57, 59, 83, 118, 124, 127, 130, 134, 158, 159, 164, 168, 174, 181
human, x, 4, 8, 10, 11, 12, 15, 19, 20, 21, 24, 26, 28, 44, 45, 48, 49, 51, 54, 56, 57, 64, 69, 73, 76, 80, 83, 111, 116, 118, 156, 159, 167, 171, 173, 183
human body, 26, 156
human health, 8, 69, 116, 171
human neutrophils, 51
human skin, 64
hygiene, 158, 162, 165, 169, 174

I

immune defense, 83
immune modulation, 34
immune response, 5, 8, 17, 19, 44, 55, 56, 57
immune system, viii, 2, 5, 7, 8, 9, 15, 19, 21, 30, 31, 83, 84
immunity, 9, 10, 19, 20, 26, 49, 50, 55, 56, 124, 134
immunocompromised, 10, 45, 87, 170
impetigo, ix, 121, 125, 126, 127, 142, 143, 146, 148
in vitro, viii, 3, 7, 10, 12, 13, 23, 24, 29, 34, 44, 61, 64, 65, 66, 69, 71, 73, 75, 96, 98, 99, 104, 114, 118, 151
in vivo, 10, 29, 32, 43, 96, 98, 99, 100, 115
incubation period, 27
individuals, 19, 33, 75, 83, 87, 108, 157, 158, 165, 166, 174, 182
infection, viii, 2, 4, 5, 7, 10, 11, 16, 19, 21, 22, 23, 24, 25, 26, 29, 32, 34, 38, 41, 42, 46, 47, 48, 52, 55, 56, 58, 59, 60, 65, 71, 81, 83, 85, 87, 88, 97, 100, 102, 104, 105, 107, 109, 110, 113, 115, 118, 120, 125, 127, 128, 129, 130, 131, 133, 134, 135, 136,148, 157, 158, 159, 160, 162, 164, 165, 166, 167, 175, 177
infective endocarditis, 81, 90, 130, 136, 137, 141, 182
inflammation, 30, 128, 134, 137
inhibition, 5, 7, 35, 38, 65, 68, 91, 92, 104, 115
injury, iv, 24, 25, 169, 184
intensive care unit, 108, 114, 130, 156, 176, 179, 183
intravenous antibiotics, 122, 137
intravenously, 29, 93, 140, 171

K

keratinocytes, 32, 64, 100

L

lactate dehydrogenase, 27
lesions, 29, 31, 125, 126
leukocytes, 136, 159
linezolid, 58, 59, 81, 84, 92, 94, 95, 104, 119, 129, 132, 133, 135, 140, 143, 144, 152, 172, 181

liposomes, iv, vii, 2, 3, 6, 7, 25, 26, 30, 42, 43, 61, 99, 100, 101, 109, 116, 117
livestock, 64, 81, 88, 111, 166, 167, 173, 174, 176, 177, 178, 180
livestock-associated MRSA (LA-MRSA), 81, 88, 111, 166, 167, 168, 174, 176, 177, 178, 181, 182
lower respiratory tract infection, 138
lysis, 5, 10, 21, 94, 124, 160

M

macrophages, 29, 62, 97, 102, 124, 159, 160
magnetic resonance, 135
magnetic resonance imaging, 135
management, 130, 135, 142, 145, 148, 151, 177
mechanical ventilation, 13, 88, 133
medical, vii, ix, 8, 70, 72, 80, 82, 98, 114, 122, 147
medical care, ix, 80
medicine, vii, viii, 2, 3, 4, 5, 6, 33, 35, 36, 37, 39, 84, 106, 144
mice, 7, 9, 10, 12, 13, 16, 30, 42, 52, 59, 62, 66, 97, 102, 113
microbiota, 7, 75, 76, 77, 84, 156
microorganism, ix, 5, 8, 31, 80, 83, 86, 103, 106
microorganisms, 4, 26, 71, 84, 96, 141, 176, 181
modern science, 66
molecular biology, 81
molecular oxygen, 30
molecular weight, 23, 101, 116
molecules, viii, 2, 9, 11, 23, 25, 27, 30, 33, 37, 38, 115, 134, 158
monoclonal antibodies (mAbs), iv, vii, 2, 3, 6, 7, 8, 9, 10, 12, 13, 14, 44, 45, 51
monoclonal antibody, 10, 11, 12, 44, 45, 46, 47, 48
mononeuritis multiplex, 70

morbidity, 81, 88, 122, 124, 157, 160
mortality, ix, 4, 10, 18, 31, 45, 80, 81, 82, 83, 86, 88, 95, 106, 108, 113, 114, 122, 124, 128, 129, 130, 133, 136, 145, 148, 151, 152, 157, 160
mortality rate, ix, 4, 18, 80, 81, 82, 83, 86, 95
MRSA infections, iv, v, vii, ix, x, 5, 7, 8, 10, 13, 19, 35, 38, 62, 80, 81, 82, 87, 88, 89, 90, 93, 94, 95, 99, 101, 102, 103, 104, 121, 122, 124, 129, 133, 156, 157, 161, 162, 163, 164, 165, 166, 167, 168, 169, 170, 171, 172, 173
mupirocin, 102, 112, 126, 127, 142, 143, 149, 152

N

nadifloxacin, 126, 127, 145, 148
nanoparticles, 26, 27, 28, 29, 61, 62, 65, 68, 76, 99, 100, 101, 109, 115, 116, 119
nanorods, 27
nanosystems, 82
nanotechnologies, 107
nanotechnology, iv, vii, viii, 2, 3, 6, 25, 26, 30, 61, 79, 98, 111
natural products, 37, 96, 98, 112
necrotizing fasciitis, 127, 128, 143, 146
neonates, 12, 47, 48, 116, 125, 160
nephrotoxicity, 131, 132
neutrophils, 5, 52, 124, 128, 159, 165
new therapy approaches., 80
non-steroidal anti-inflammatory drugs, 103, 107
nosocomial infections, 14, 119, 129, 156, 157, 180
nosocomial pneumonia, 92
nucleic acid, viii, 2, 20, 21, 33

O

obesity, 75, 138
oil, 37, 65, 68, 101, 110
optical density, 36
optical parameters, 65
oral antibiotic, ix, 121, 122, 128, 135
oral antibiotics, 122, 128, 135
oral cavity, 20
organism, 34, 122, 123, 124, 136
organs, 4, 12, 29, 38, 83, 97
osteomyelitis, 24, 25, 60, 80, 90, 130, 134, 135, 136, 140, 145, 150, 151, 156, 159, 173, 177
oxazolidinones, 92, 109, 117

P

pain, 3, 128, 129, 133, 136
penicillin, x, 4, 7, 10, 18, 81, 85, 86, 90, 92, 106, 112, 114, 116, 117, 123, 138, 155, 156, 161
peptide, 6, 28, 94, 105, 110, 123
peripheral blood, 10
peripheral blood mononuclear cell, 10
peritonitis, 10, 96, 97
permeability, 28, 38
personal hygiene, 158, 165, 168, 169
phage, 21, 23, 24, 25, 57, 58, 59, 117
pharmaceutical, 26, 96, 107, 115, 120
pharmacokinetics, 11, 12, 45, 46, 48, 117
photodynamic therapy, vii, viii, 2, 43, 64, 65
photodynamic therapy (PDT), iv, vii, viii, 2, 3, 7, 30, 31, 32, 43, 63, 64, 65
photosensitizers, 30, 31
physical properties, 98
physicochemical properties, 25
placebo, 11, 12, 13, 18, 33, 46, 47, 48, 54, 65, 146
plants, 36, 96, 169, 181, 182

pneumonia, ix, 12, 13, 14, 16, 20, 24, 25, 45, 48, 52, 55, 80, 81, 86, 88, 90, 92, 94, 116, 121, 130, 133, 140, 141, 142, 150, 151, 156, 164, 165, 172, 173, 179
polysaccharides, 5, 6, 15, 18, 51, 84
population, viii, x, 2, 20, 22, 56, 116, 142, 155, 156, 157, 158, 166, 167, 173
prevention, 3, 5, 7, 8, 10, 11, 36, 38, 47, 48, 97, 100, 114, 119, 149
prosthetic device, 156, 158
protection, 7, 8, 10, 16, 19, 24, 42, 52, 55, 59, 113
protein synthesis, 90, 92, 103
proteins, viii, 2, 6, 18, 21, 23, 27, 28, 30, 31, 32, 33, 37, 81, 103, 124, 137, 158, 159
public health, vii, 2, 4, 31, 82, 156, 173

R

reactive oxygen, 6, 27, 30, 32, 63, 104
receptor, 6, 21, 52, 159
researchers, 8, 13, 26, 28, 29, 97
resistance, ix, x, 4, 20, 23, 31, 34, 37, 38, 40, 64, 80, 81, 82, 85, 86, 88, 89, 92, 93, 95, 96, 103, 104, 105, 106, 108, 109, 115, 121, 122, 123, 126, 131, 132, 133, 135, 136, 142, 143, 144, 145, 147, 149, 155, 156, 161, 164, 168, 170, 171, 173, 175, 176, 177, 178, 184
resolution, 31, 93, 126, 130
resources, 36, 40, 88, 157
respiration, 28
response, 5, 12, 15, 19, 31, 34, 83, 97, 113, 127, 130
retail, 167, 176, 177, 178
retapumulin, 127
risk, ix, 4, 10, 12, 19, 34, 80, 87, 88, 89, 95, 107, 114, 117, 133, 135, 137, 149, 156, 158, 159, 165, 166, 167, 168, 169, 171, 172, 173, 177, 178

risk factors, ix, 80, 87, 88, 107, 133, 137, 169

S

safety, 10, 11, 12, 13, 17, 46, 47, 48, 60, 94, 146, 148
sepsis, 11, 16, 47, 48, 83, 97, 118, 130, 156, 164
septic arthritis, 130, 134, 136, 158
skin, ix, x, 16, 19, 20, 24, 31, 32, 64, 81, 82, 83, 93, 100, 116, 121, 124, 125, 126, 127, 128, 129, 130, 138, 140, 141, 144, 145, 148, 155, 156, 158, 160, 164, 165, 166, 168, 169, 170, 172, 173, 175, 179
skin and soft tissue infections, 93, 124, 172
society, 115, 131, 147, 174, 179
species, 6, 20, 23, 26, 30, 32, 34, 36, 118, 161, 166, 167
staphylococci, 102, 108, 113, 114, 138, 144
Staphylococcus aureus, iv, v, vi, vii, ix, x, 1, 2, 3, 4, 8, 12, 23, 24, 25, 26, 29, 31, 37, 40, 41, 42, 43, 44, 45, 46, 47, 48, 49, 50, 51, 52, 53, 54, 55, 56, 57, 58, 59, 60, 61, 62, 63, 64, 65, 67, 68, 79, 80, 82, 84, 85, 86, 90, 106, 107, 108, 109, 110, 111, 112, 113, 114, 115, 116, 117, 118, 119, 121, 122, 140, 141, 142, 143, 144, 145, 146, 147, 148, 149, 150, 151, 152, 155, 156, 158, 159, 161, 162, 165, 168, 170, 171, 174, 175, 176, 177, 178, 179, 180, 181, 182, 183, 184
structure, 23, 31, 34, 53, 74, 103, 130, 138, 140, 141, 172, 173
sulphamethoxazole-trimethoprim, 122, 126, 128
surface component, 11, 134, 158
surfactant, 29, 90, 99, 132, 151, 172
surgical intervention, 135
surgical site infections, 124, 128, 129, 142, 148, 149, 152

surveillance, 40, 130, 157, 162, 175, 184
susceptibility, ix, 8, 19, 26, 35, 56, 66, 80, 81, 82, 84, 103, 107, 112, 114, 138, 139, 152, 172
symptoms, vii, x, 12, 13, 33, 122, 130, 133, 137, 156
syndrome, 6, 83, 116, 125, 160
synergistic effect, 29, 102, 103, 104, 107, 114, 171
synthesis, 31, 89, 91, 94, 103, 123, 126, 127, 161

T

teicoplanin, 91, 94, 108, 114, 116, 129, 135
temperature, 159, 166
therapeutic approaches, vii, ix, 80, 82
therapeutic effect, 28, 31, 93, 95, 106
therapeutic effects, 93
therapeutic use, 67
therapeutics, viii, 3, 46, 112, 174
therapy, ix, 3, 6, 7, 8, 10, 11, 13, 20, 23, 24, 25, 26, 28, 30, 31, 37, 43, 46, 48, 49, 57, 58, 59, 60, 61, 63, 80, 88, 89, 92, 95, 97, 100, 103, 104, 108, 110, 111, 119, 127, 129, 131, 133, 135, 136, 137, 138, 139, 146, 151, 159, 171, 173, 179, 181
tissue, 5, 7, 81, 83, 90, 93, 124, 128, 137, 144, 148, 156, 158, 159, 160, 165, 166, 169, 172, 173, 175
toxic shock syndrome, 18, 53, 83, 115, 159, 165, 175
toxicity, 10, 25, 30, 37, 92, 95, 98, 142
toxin, 6, 12, 14, 17, 18, 45, 48, 124, 125, 150, 159, 160, 183
transmission, x, 83, 118, 156, 162, 165, 166, 167, 168, 169, 173, 180, 183
treatment, vii, viii, ix, x, 2, 3, 4, 5, 7, 8, 9, 10, 11, 13, 26, 27, 30, 31, 32, 33, 35, 36, 38, 39, 42, 43, 45, 46, 48, 58, 60, 80, 81, 82, 84, 86, 88, 89, 90, 92, 93, 94, 95, 96,

Index

100, 101, 102, 103, 104, 106, 109, 112, 114, 115, 116, 117, 118, 119, 120, 121, 125, 126, 128, 129, 130, 131, 132, 135, 137, 138, 139, 140, 141, 142, 143, 145, 146, 147, 148, 152, 156, 169, 171, 172, 173, 177, 179, 181, 182

trial, 11, 12, 13, 15, 17, 45, 47, 53, 54, 60, 70, 76, 96, 146

U

United Kingdom, 86, 87, 123, 157, 162, 170, 178
United Nations, 40
United States, 4, 41, 87, 157, 175, 179, 181, 182
upper respiratory tract, 156
urinary tract, 20, 165, 172
urinary tract infection, 165, 172

V

vaccine, viii, 2, 15, 16, 17, 18, 19, 20, 41, 42, 49, 50, 51, 52, 53, 54, 55, 56, 57, 107

vaccines, iv, vii, 2, 3, 6, 7, 15, 16, 19, 20, 49, 50, 51, 52, 53, 54, 55, 82
valvular heart disease, 137
vancomycin, ix, 7, 12, 13, 28, 29, 43, 48, 62, 80, 81, 84, 89, 90, 92, 93, 94, 95, 98, 99, 101, 104, 105, 109, 110, 111, 112, 113, 116, 119, 122, 129, 131, 132, 133, 135, 138, 139, 140, 141, 142, 144, 147, 150, 152, 153, 164, 171, 172, 173, 182
vancomycin-intermediate *S. aureus* (VISA), 82, 89, 97, 132, 171
vancomycin-resistant *S. aureus* (VRSA), ix, 80, 82, 89, 110, 132

W

workers, 157, 162, 165, 168, 169, 176, 180
worldwide, vii, ix, 2, 4, 20, 80, 86, 183
wound healing, 31, 43, 63
wound infection, 24, 101, 164